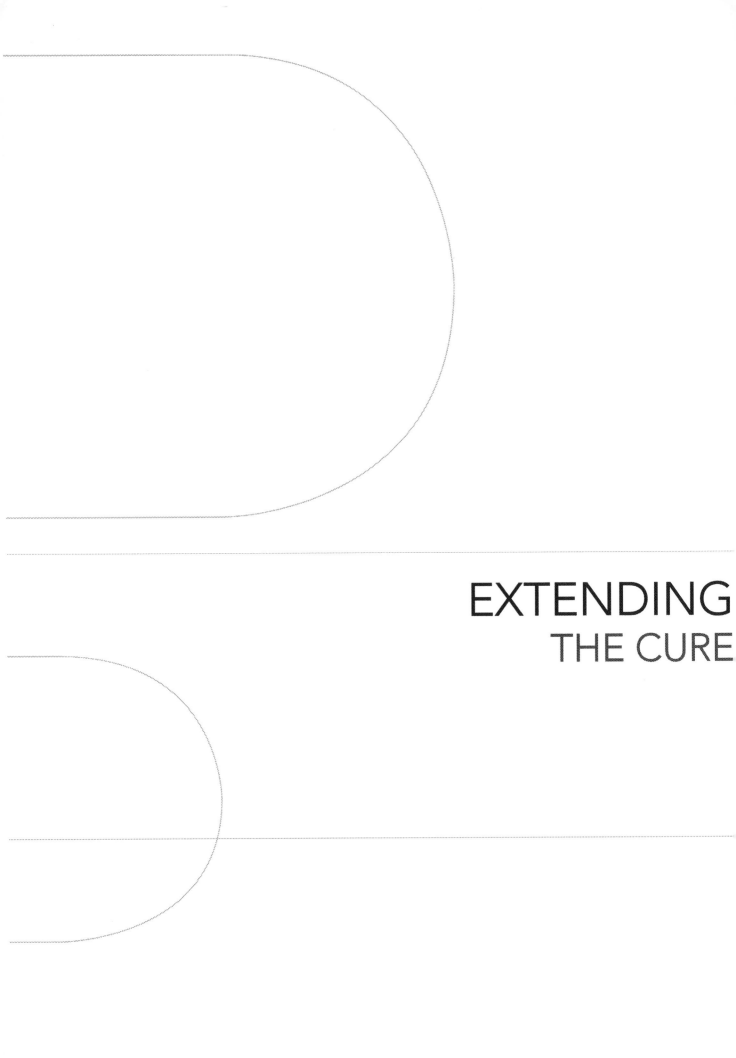

# EXTENDING
## THE CURE

**RAMANAN LAXMINARAYAN** and **ANUP MALANI**

with David Howard and David L. Smith

# EXTENDING
## THE CURE

Policy responses to the growing threat of antibiotic resistance

**LIBRARY OF CONGRESS CATALOGING-IN-PUBLICATION DATA**

Laxminarayan, Ramanan.

Extending the cure : policy responses to the growing threat of antibiotic resistance / by Ramanan Laxminarayan and Anup Malani ; with David Howard and David L. Smith.

p. ; cm.

Includes bibliographical references.

ISBN 978-1-933115-57-3 (pbk. : alk. Paper)  1.  Drug resistance in microorganisms—United States. 2.  Drug resistance in microorganisms—Government policy—United States.

I. Malani, Anup. II. Title. III. Title: Policy responses to the growing threat of antibiotic resistance.

[DNLM: 1.  Drug Resistance, Bacterial—United States. 2.  Anti-Bacterial Agents—United States. 3.  Drug Utilization—United States. 4.  Health Policy—United States.  QW 52 L425e 2007]

QR177.L39 2007

616.9`041—dc22                                                                                             2007008949

**RESOURCES FOR THE FUTURE**

1616 P Street, NW
Washington, DC 20036-1400
USA
www.rff.org

**ABOUT RESOURCES FOR THE FUTURE**

RFF is a nonprofit and nonpartisan organization that conducts independent research—rooted primarily in economics and other social sciences—on environmental, energy, natural resources, and public health issues. RFF is headquartered in Washington, D.C., but its research scope comprises programs in nations around the world. Founded in 1952, RFF pioneered the application of economics as a tool to develop more effective policy for the use and conservation of natural resources. Its scholars employ social science methods to analyze critical issues concerning antibiotic and antimalarial resistance, pollution control, energy policy, land and water use, hazardous waste, climate change, and the environmental and health challenges of developing countries.

**DISCLAIMER**

The statements in this book represent the opinions of the authors; the statements do not and should not be construed to represent official policy statements or endorsements by Resources for the Future, the Robert Wood Johnson Foundation, the Fogarty International Center, the National Institutes of Health, the Department of Health and Human Services, or the U.S. federal government.

What does not destroy me makes me stronger.

—*Nietzsche, 1899*

It is not difficult to make microbes resistant to penicillin in the laboratory by exposing them to concentrations not sufficient to kill them, and the same thing has occasionally happened in the body…

—*Alexander Fleming, 1945*

# Contents

## THE EXTENDING THE CURE PROJECT

This report was prepared by a team led by Ramanan Laxminarayan and comprising Anup Malani, David Howard, and David L. Smith, Eili Klein, and Sarah Darley. An advisory committee chaired by Kenneth J. Arrow and comprising Donald Kennedy, Simon A. Levin, Saul Levmore, and John E. McGowan, Jr., provided valuable guidance at all stages of the report's preparation.

Preparation of this report was immensely aided by the contributions of participants in a series of consultations; the names of participants are listed at the end of this report. The team also received useful input at various stages of the research process from Judy Cahill, Neil Fishman, Clarissa Long, Dean Lueck, Sharlene Matten, Tom Nachbar, Dennis O'Leary, Bill Sage, and Robert Wise. John Bartlett, Ed Belongia, Carl Bergstrom, Marty Blaser, Barry Eisenstein, Neil Fishman, Eric Kades, Keith Klugman, Lou Rice, Ed Septimus, Brad Spellberg, and Jim Wilen provided helpful reviews on the final draft. Report review by infectious disease experts was coordinated by the Infectious Diseases Society of America. Consultation participants and reviewers provided substantive and valuable input to the report, but they were not asked to endorse its conclusions and did not see the final version before it was published. The authors bear full responsibility for the final content.

Eili Klein provided extensive substantive input, including preparation of graphs, tables, and text boxes for the report. Sarah Darley coordinated logistics for the consultations and overall report production. Hellen Gelband, Piper Kerman, and Ed Walz provided significant input on the executive summary. The report was edited by Sally Atwater, Felicia Day and Sarah Beam.

The **Extending the Cure** project and this report were made possible by financial support from the Robert Wood Johnson Foundation's Pioneer Portfolio.

# Foreword

Few public health developments present greater challenges to modern society than the growing resistance of many infectious diseases to antibiotics. In a sense, medical research has become a victim of its own success: creating wonder drugs that heal millions yet could be rendered obsolete through sheer overuse.

At a time when cases of drug-resistant infections continue to accumulate, Extending the Cure provides a rational and clear strategy to deal with this impending crisis—and policymakers would be wise to heed the advice before it is too late.

In this report, Ramanan Laxminarayan and his colleagues suggest a range of efforts that can restructure incentives and lead to significant changes in how patients, doctors, hospitals, and drug companies regard and use antibiotics. There is a role for insurance companies in employing reimbursement methods that do not encourage overuse of antibiotics. There is a role for physicians and medical associations to adopt standards that would discourage inappropriate antibiotic use. And there is a clear role for government—to promote careful demonstration projects, including providing incentives, to push hospitals to engage in better infection control and pharmaceutical makers to boost antibiotic research. Just as important, public awareness campaigns are needed to educate parents, doctors, clinics, and patients about the threat of drug-resistant infections.

From my 20 years of service on the House Energy and Commerce Committee, which has jurisdiction over health matters, I know how critical it is to have information that has been thoroughly analyzed and vetted. The authors of this report have carried out a vital first step, assessing the array of policy options, and providing a range of practical options for consideration. Of course, genuine change will only come from public pressure and political compromise, but Extending the Cure offers a long-overdue assessment of options for a successful policy outcome.

Resources for the Future is grateful to the members of the Extending the Cure Advisory Committee, who provided valuable guidance, and to the Robert Wood Johnson Foundation for its commitment to support this important research.

**PHILIP SHARP**

*President,* Resources for the Future

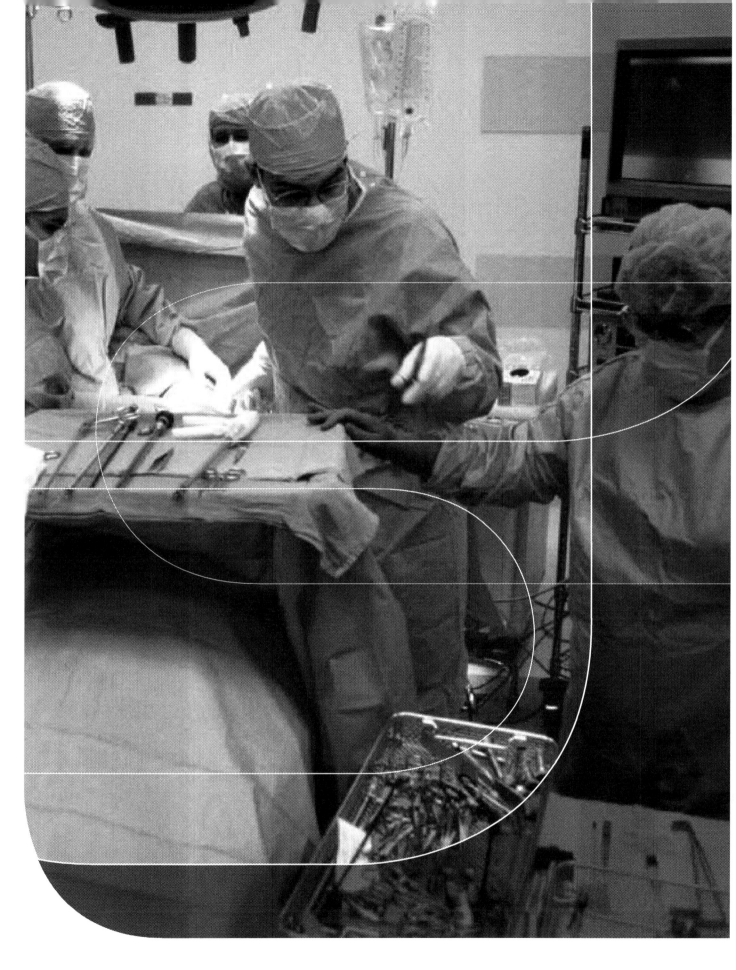

# Executive Summary

Modern medicine depends on effective antibiotics to control bacterial infections. Since the first of these wonder drugs appeared a mere 65 years ago, they have transformed the practice of medicine and saved millions of lives. But today, at the start of the 21st century, the rapid rate of emergence and spread of bacterial pathogens resistant to antibiotics threatens to return us to an era when common infections were untreatable.

The growing problem of antibiotic-resistant *Staphylococcus aureus* (*S. aureus* or "staph") is illustrative (Figure ES.1). In 1987, 2 percent of patients infected with *S. aureus* failed to respond to methicillin, an inexpensive antibiotic that had been effective against these infections since the 1960s. By 2004, more than 50 percent of patients with *S. aureus* failed to respond to methicillin, with terrible consequences. Already a few cases of resistance to vancomycin, the drug often used to treat MRSA infections, have been reported.

*Streptococcus pneumoniae* (*S. pneumoniae*), another common pathogen, causes bacterial meningitis and bacterial pneumonia, among other conditions. In 1987, only 2 of every 10,000 *S. pneumoniae* infections—0.02 percent—were resistant to penicillin, the antibiotic of choice. By 2004, this figure had risen to 1 in 5—20 percent—a 1,000-fold increase (CDC 2005).

According to the U.S. Food and Drug Administration (FDA), "Unless antibiotic resistance problems are detected as they emerge, and actions are taken to contain them, the world could be faced with previously treatable diseases that have again become untreatable, as in the days before antibiotics were developed" (Interagency Task Force on Antimicrobial Resistance 2001). Major reports in recent years have called for steps to address this growing threat before it engulfs the medical system (ASM 1994; OTA 1995; Harrison and Lederberg 1998), yet policymakers have taken astonishingly little action.

Antibiotic effectiveness can be thought of as a natural resource, much like oil, fish, or forests (Laxminarayan and Brown 2001;

> ## "The world could be faced with previously treatable diseases that have again become untreatable..."
>
> — Interagency Task Force on Antimicrobial Resistance

Laxminarayan 2003): it is a resource accessible to anyone who can purchase it. All antibiotic use, appropriate or not, "uses up" some of the effectiveness of that antibiotic, diminishing our ability to use it in the future. Hastening the spread of resistance by overuse of antibiotics is like other shared resource problems, such as global warming or overfishing—a phenomenon referred to as "the tragedy of the commons" (Hardin 1968). Approaching antibiotic resistance as a resource

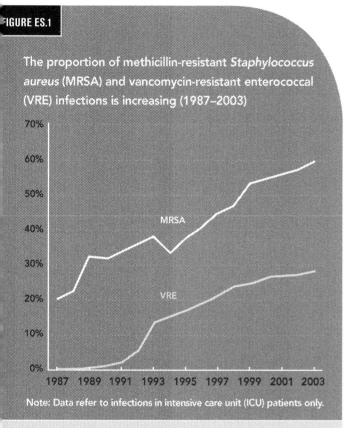

**FIGURE ES.1**

The proportion of methicillin-resistant *Staphylococcus aureus* (MRSA) and vancomycin-resistant enterococcal (VRE) infections is increasing (1987–2003)

Note: Data refer to infections in intensive care unit (ICU) patients only.

**Sources:** VRE and MRSA data, 1998–2000, 2002–2003 (CDC 1999; CDC 2000; CDC 2001; CDC 2003; CDC 2004); data for 2001 are the average of 2000 and 2002 data. MRSA data from 1987–1997 are estimated from (Lowy 1998). VRE data for 1989 and 1993 are from (CDC 1993). VRE data for 1990–1992 and 1994–1997 are interpolated based on geometric mean.

existing antibiotics, sensibly encourage the discovery of new antibiotics, and give drug companies a greater incentive to sell these new drugs responsibly. The policy changes considered here go beyond simply tinkering with the current system; instead, we address deep weaknesses in how we develop, regulate, and manage antibiotics.

The report is the result of a two-year study by researchers at Resources for the Future, the University of Chicago, the National Institutes of Health, and Emory University. It objectively evaluates a range of policy options for dealing with antibiotic resistance. The policy options presented here were debated at four consultations with medical and scientific experts who provided invaluable insights into the incentives behind choices concerning antibiotic use and development. The research focused on antibiotic use in medicine and did not explicitly address the problem of antibiotic overuse in agriculture for growth promotion, but clearly it is important to change incentives for how the drugs are used in that context as well.

A significant finding of this work is that we lack much of the information necessary to properly evaluate these policy options, prioritize them, or combine them in effective and efficient ways. It is important to distinguish policies, the subject of this report, from techniques—that is, the actual practices, such as multidrug treatment and infection control measures in hospitals—about which more is known. The policy options involve ensuring that these effective practices are followed. The full range of policy options considered in the study, with their pros and cons and the actors involved, is summarized in Table 8.1.

The second phase of the Extending the Cure project will expand the policy research and dialogue over the next few years. Filling in these knowledge gaps should allow us to develop a comprehensive playbook of incentive-based policy options that government officials and other policymakers can use to make a real difference in the fight against antibiotic resistance.

problem is not just a convenient metaphor; it can help shape incentive-altering strategies to use antibiotics in ways that provide the greatest benefit to society, both today and in the future. Such incentives would encourage pharmaceutical companies to develop new antibiotics, and patients and health care providers to use existing antibiotics sustainably.

In this report, we examine the problem of antibiotic resistance from a natural resources perspective and propose solutions from an incentive-based perspective. Our purpose is to evaluate policy options that will enable society to make the best use of

## Antibiotic resistance and its spread

Antibiotic-resistant bacteria are a natural consequence of antibiotic use, but development and spread of these pathogens can be hastened or slowed by the way antibiotics are used. Antibiotic-resistant bacteria arise as the natural result of mutation and natural selection within a population of organisms—say, an infection in a human host—faced with an agent that eliminates most of its members. Those that survive because of mutations that circumvent the effect of the antibiotic (through a variety of mechanisms) can multiply and give rise to larger numbers of antibiotic-resistant bacteria. In the absence of alternative antibiotics or other control mechanisms, these antibiotic-resistant bacteria can spread to other people just like any other bacterial infection (for example, through personal contact or inhalation of droplets from coughing). If they are robust enough, they can become widespread. Complicating matters, in many cases bacteria acquire resistance to antibiotics through the transfer of genetic material from other species of bacteria. In addition, resistance to one antibiotic may confer resistance to related antibiotics.

Antibiotic resistance cannot be prevented. Every time antibiotics are used, whether they save a life or are used to no effect (to treat viral rather than bacterial infections, for example), the effective lifespan of that antibiotic and perhaps related drugs is shortened. The tension between individual good and collective good is central to the issue. The average patient suffering from a cold or an ear infection wants immediate relief and sees a prescription for antibiotics as the ticket to recovery, and the physician may be only too

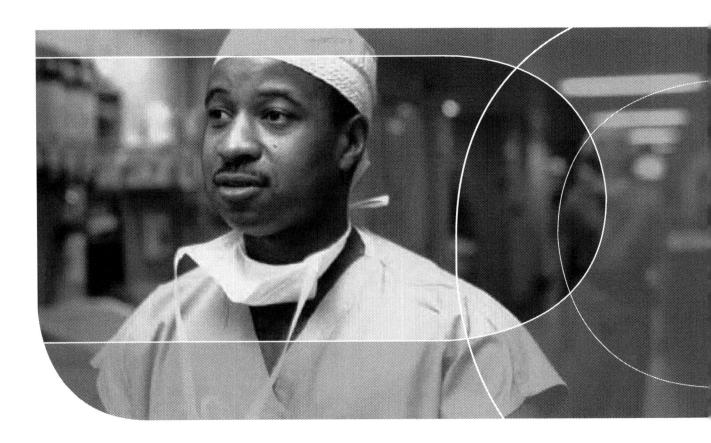

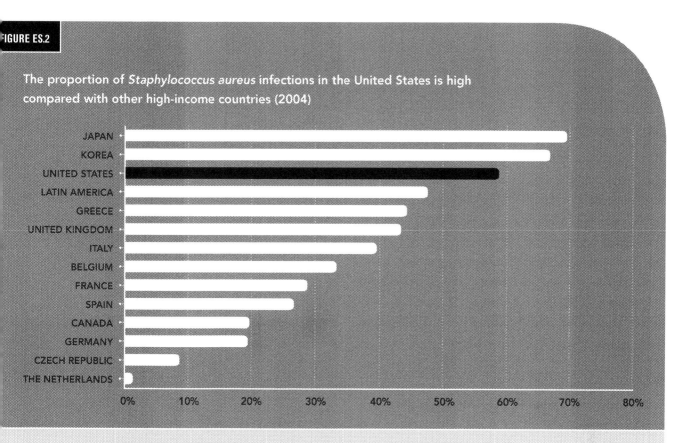

The proportion of *Staphylococcus aureus* infections in the United States is high compared with other high-income countries (2004)

**Sources:** United States (Jones, Draghi et al. 2004), Japan (Bell and Turnidge 2002), Korea (Lee, Kim et al. 2004), Latin America (Diekema, Pfaller et al. 2000), European countries (RIVM 2005).

happy to oblige if writing it benefits her practice. Neither may consider that antibiotic use by one patient eventually reduces the drug's effectiveness for everyone.

Hospitals, too, ignore the larger context of their response to infection, particularly hospital-acquired infection, by preferring treatment over prevention. Antibiotics are often less expensive than other forms of infection control, and hospitals can even pass off the costs of antibiotic treatment to managed-care providers. Compounding the problem, hospitals have no incentive to ensure that the patients they discharge are not carrying a resistant pathogen from their facilities to other health care institutions.

Although pharmaceutical companies, the makers of antibiotics, have a profit motive to consider the effect of resistance on the antibiotics they own, other firms may have drugs that work in similar ways. Just as many farmers drawing water from the same aquifer have no incentive to care about how fast the aquifer is being depleted, no one firm needs to care about resistance because the burden of resistance as it relates to the lifespan of salable antibiotics is borne by all firms.

The barriers to addressing the problem of antibiotic resistance all involve conflict between the interest of individual decisionmakers and the interest of society as a whole, now and in the future. Incentive-based policy solutions can help patients, physicians, hospitals, and pharmaceutical companies consider the impact of their decisions on others and give them the opportunity to help the solution evolve.

The phenomenon of antibiotic resistance has been anticipated since the introduction of penicillin. The search for new antibiotics was always aimed at more effective products, but also with the recognition that older drugs would be lost to resistance and new ones would be needed. Early on, the potential for new and better antibiotics might have seemed limitless. Today, the need for them is urgent. The challenge—the subject of this report—is how to change the incentives of all the actors and thereby maximize the useful lifespan of today's antibiotics and those still to be developed.

■

## Antibiotic resistance in the United States: status and impact

More than 63,000 patients in the United States die every year from hospital-acquired bacterial infections that are resistant to at least one common antibiotic (Gerberding 2003)—more deaths than from AIDS, traffic accidents, or influenza. The number may actually be higher because many deaths attributed to other causes, particularly those of elderly patients suffering from multiple conditions, may in reality be due to antibiotic-resistant infections.

:: COMPARISON WITH OTHER COUNTRIES

Some of the most serious and widespread antibiotic-resistance problems worldwide are infections caused by MRSA and vancomycin-resistant enterococci (VRE). Data on the prevalence of these infections are available from many countries around the world, and the United States does not compare favorably.

About half of all patients treated in intensive care units for *S. aureus* in U.S. hospitals cannot be treated with methicillin or older antibiotics (CDC 2004), a much higher proportion than in most other high-income countries (Figure ES.2). Spreading resistance combined with an increasing number of *S. aureus* infections has resulted in a growing number of hospitalized patients who have MRSA infections (Figure ES.3).

U.S. hospitals also rank high in infections from species of the bacteria genus *Enterococcus* that are resistant to vancomycin—one of the most powerful antibiotics available. More than 12 percent of enteroccocal infections in U.S. hospitals are

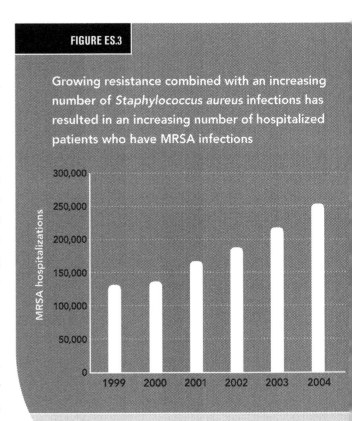

**FIGURE ES.3**

Growing resistance combined with an increasing number of *Staphylococcus aureus* infections has resulted in an increasing number of hospitalized patients who have MRSA infections

MRSA hospitalizations

**Source:** The Surveillance Network (TSN) Database-USA (Focus Technologies, Herndon, VA, USA).

resistant to vancomycin, with even higher rates in intensive care units (McDonald 2006). In Europe, only Portugal reports a higher proportion of VRE infections.

## :: ECONOMIC IMPACT OF ANTIBIOTIC-RESISTANT INFECTIONS

In addition to their death toll, drug-resistant infections impose a significant financial cost on patients, health care systems, and society. The annual additional cost of treating hospital-acquired infections from just six species of antibiotic-resistant bacteria was estimated to be at least $1.3 billion in 1992 dollars ($1.87 billion in 2006 dollars)—more than annual spending on influenza (OTA 1995; AHRQ 2003). The Pennsylvania Health Care Cost Containment Commission estimated that during 2004, at least $20 billion was billed nationally to Medicare for hospital-acquired infections, many of which were resistant to one or more classes of antibiotics.

Many studies have documented longer hospital stays and increased costs for medication and care associated with resistant infections. The situation where an infection does not respond to any known antibiotic is becoming increasingly common. Since death or serious disabilities are likely outcomes, the future costs of multidrug-resistant strains are only going to increase.

Another significant cost of drug resistance comes from periodic switches to newer, more expensive antibiotics. As the risk of treatment failure increases, the entire system must shift to new drugs even if older drugs retain some effectiveness. Whereas penicillin costs pennies a dose, the newest antibiotics can run a few thousand dollars for a course of treatment. Even with modest levels of resistance to antibiotics, patients have to be dosed with two or more drugs to ensure successful treatment. As a result, for example, increased drug resistance has raised the annual national cost of treating ear infections by an estimated 20 percent, or $216 million (Howard and Rask 2002).

The expense of more powerful antibiotics affects the cost

> More than 63,000 patients in the United States die every year from hospital-acquired bacterial infections.

of not only treating infections but also preventing them. Modern medical practices—including all types of surgery, organ transplants, and cancer chemotherapy—involve using antibiotics to protect patients with other serious conditions, many of whom have temporarily or permanently impaired immune systems, from the added risks of serious infection. Because antibiotics are an important complement to other medical technologies, the higher cost (or diminished effectiveness) of antibiotics raises the price of other medical technologies and may imperil them if effective antibiotics are lost.

## :: MEASURING THE COSTS OF RESISTANCE

Quantifying the health and economic impacts of resistance is a significant research challenge, but it can be accomplished with the appropriate level of effort. To date, no reliable estimates of both the costs and the benefits of antibiotics in the hospital and community setting have been made. In hospitals, where antibiotic-resistant pathogens are often transmitted, one challenge is disentangling the effect of drug-resistant infections on the length of hospital stay: a hospital-acquired infection with a resistant pathogen increases the length of stay, and a longer stay increases the risk of acquiring such an infection. In community settings, the challenge is accurately estimating both the benefits and the costs of antibiotic use. Resistance-related costs alone are insufficient reasons to recommend that fewer antibiotics be used, since antibiotics have infection control benefits: they prevent the spread of susceptible pathogens.

## Overview of policy options

The potential policy options presented in this report involve all possible participants and all incentive-based tools that might be brought to bear in a comprehensive strategy for the near- and long-term stewardship of antibiotics in health care. What is missing is the information needed to evaluate each option fully and hence the ability to rank them according to cost-effectiveness or economic efficiency. We therefore present them as starting points for discussion and as the basis of a future research agenda.

An overall strategy to maintain the effectiveness of existing antibiotics for as long as possible and to encourage the development of new antibiotics would have five components:

- discouraging inappropriate antibiotic use by changing how patients are reimbursed for antibiotic prescriptions and how physicians are paid for prescribing them;
- lessening the need for some uses of antibiotics by improving infection control and vaccinating against common infections;
- designing antibiotic use strategies, such as hospital formularies, combination therapies, and cycling, that delay the emergence of resistance;
- encouraging research and development into new antibiotics; and
- reducing incentives for pharmaceutical manufacturers to oversell their antibiotics.

Those five tactics, three that reduce demand and two that address supply, are not mutually exclusive. Partial solutions to the antibiotic resistance problem—those that focus only on supply or only on demand—are likely to be less effective in the long term than solutions that are mindful of their interrelatedness. Efforts to protect new antibiotics from bacterial resistance by keeping them on the sidelines, for example, potentially reduce incentives for new drug development by the pharmaceutical industry. Yet having a supply of new antibiotics that are fundamentally different from existing ones expands treatment options and lowers the likelihood that resistance to other drugs will evolve and spread.

## Demand-side solutions: extending the therapeutic life of existing drugs

Few new antibiotics are in the development pipeline, so increasing the useful life of existing drugs must be an immediate priority. Several kinds of policies could help extend the useful therapeutic life of existing antibiotics.

- One set of policies focuses on reducing antibiotic prescribing by educating patients and physicians of the risks of greater antibiotic use and by changing incentives for health care providers and patients.
- Another set of policies reduces the need for antibiotics by lowering the burden of infections, using vaccinations in community settings and infection control in health care facilities.

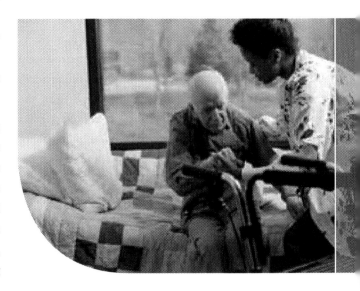

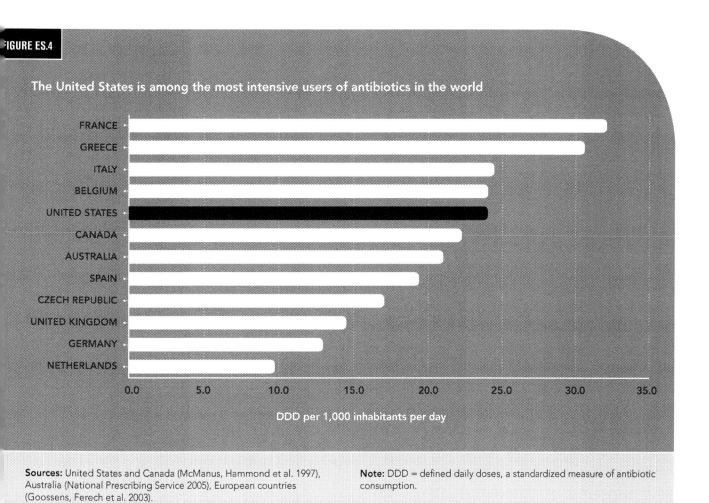

**FIGURE ES.4**

**The United States is among the most intensive users of antibiotics in the world**

DDD per 1,000 inhabitants per day

**Sources:** United States and Canada (McManus, Hammond et al. 1997), Australia (National Prescribing Service 2005), European countries (Goossens, Ferech et al. 2003).

**Note:** DDD = defined daily doses, a standardized measure of antibiotic consumption.

- A third set of policies relies on a better understanding of strategies, such as cycling, combination therapies, and antibiotic heterogeneity, to delay the emergence and spread of resistance.

## :: REDUCING ANTIBIOTIC PRESCRIBING

Lowering antibiotic use is critical to slowing the evolution of resistance. Rates of antibiotic prescribing in the United States are among the highest in the world (Figure ES.4). Reducing prescribing, however, involves a tension between what is good for the individual patient and what is good for the rest of society. Patient and physician education can decrease antibiotic use to some degree, but the long-term effectiveness of educational programs is unclear.

## :: REDUCING THE NEED FOR ANTIBIOTICS

**Vaccination in the community.** Vaccinations can lower the incidence of infections and thus the need for antibiotics, and this approach is immediately feasible. A policy of routinely vaccinating children against pneumococci, for instance, would reduce the number of infections. It is not currently mandatory, however, and it is relatively expensive. A national requirement for childhood pneumococcal vaccinations and a lower vaccine price could greatly reduce the need for antibiotics in children under the age of five, who consume a significant proportion of antibiotics used in the community. A vaccine to prevent MRSA infections could lower the need for antibiotics in health care facilities but is not yet available. Federal support of research on an MRSA vaccine may be useful in expediting vaccine development.

**Infection control in hospitals.** Containing bacterial infections in community settings will require significant time and resources, but relatively immediate infection control in health care facilities can be highly effective (and cost saving). Hospitals are focal points for the evolution of resistance because most hospital patients are administered antibiotics, and patients carrying a resistant strain are rapidly discharged—stays average just five days in U.S. hospitals (DeFrances, Hall et al. 2005)—and replaced with noncarriers. Infection control can therefore be very effective at reducing transmission within the hospital. Today, however, hospitals and long-term care facilities are reluctant to invest in practices that would reduce transmission—such as isolating incoming patients colonized with a resistant infection, encouraging hand washing and consistent use of caps and gowns, and changing staff cohorting (assigning nursing staff to a small number of patients to prevent wider contact)—because it is less expensive to use antibiotics.

Two other factors may affect hospitals' decisions to invest in infection control. One is financial: the costs of staff time and equipment purchased for infection control are borne by the hospital, whereas antibiotics are covered by health insurers. The other involves "free-riding:" because patients use more than one hospital, each institution has an incentive to take advantage of the infection control efforts of others while not making the investment itself, and consequently overall

levels of infection with resistant strains remain high. Where infection control programs operate at a regional level—as in the Netherlands, for example—all hospitals share both the costs and the benefits of better infection control.

## :: USING INNOVATIVE TREATMENT STRATEGIES

Ecological understanding can be applied to formulate antibiotic use strategies to lower the likelihood of resistance development. Strategies such as using drug combinations and cycling of antibiotics (similar to pesticide rotation in agriculture to delay the development of pesticide-resistant insects) have been proposed but have not been rigorously evaluated. A strategy of treating different patients who have the same type of infection with fundamentally different antibiotics has been proposed to slow the spread of resistance, but it remains to be tested widely.

■

## Supply-side solutions: encouraging development of new antibiotics

Even if we were to make the best use of existing drugs, resistance would arise. However, in recent decades the development of new antibiotics has not kept pace with resistance. Investment in antibiotics appears to be declining (Figure ES.5) and new antibiotic development has been limited mainly to addressing MRSA. While MRSA is a significant health risk, new antibiotics are needed to combat infections caused by Gram-negative organisms, where resistance is rising rapidly.

## :: ENCOURAGING NEW ANTIBIOTICS

Policies to encourage development of new antibiotics that have been contemplated so far include tax incentives for research spending, patent extensions for other drugs in a pharmaceutical company's portfolio in exchange for developing a new antibiotic ("wild card" patent extensions), and liability protection from the adverse side effects of new

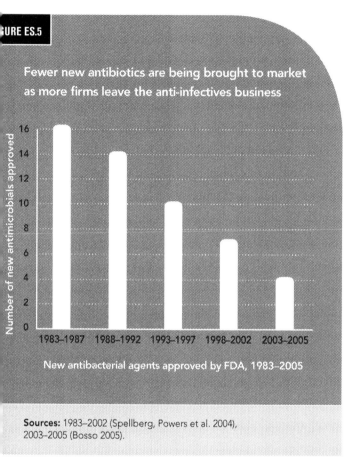

**Sources:** 1983–2002 (Spellberg, Powers et al. 2004),
2003–2005 (Bosso 2005).

of an antibiotic today could diminish the effectiveness of new drugs in the pipeline if they work in similar ways or are chemically related. For this reason, patents alone do not give pharmaceutical firms an incentive to care about resistance. Further, many antibiotics are off patent and manufactured by more than one company, each of which has an incentive to sell as much as possible.

Solving the problem of "who owns antibiotic effectiveness" is a significant challenge. Options include revisions of U.S. patent law to create a new, patent-like marketing right (similar in concept to market exclusivity under the Orphan Drug Act) and antitrust exemptions that would enable different antibiotic patent holders to work together to prevent the emergence of resistance.

## Federal stewardship of antibiotic effectiveness

Antibiotic effectiveness (in contrast to the antibiotics themselves) is a shared resource, like clean air or safe drinking water. Because it is not owned by any single entity, markets are unlikely to result in sustainable antibiotic use. Private markets may not be able to induce higher levels of infection control or appropriate antibiotic use, but government might.

A useful precedent for government intervention to protect against resistance is the successful effort by the Environmental Protection Agency (EPA) to prevent the emergence of pesticide-resistant agricultural pests. EPA currently regulates bioengineered crops, such as corn with transgenic *Bacillus thuringiensis* (*Bt*), and requires that farmers grow traditional crops in "refuges" that can harbor susceptible pests and thereby delay the emergence of resistance to the bioengineered variety. These policies have been in place since the mid-1990s, and thus far, no resistance to *Bt* crops has been detected.

But for resistance to antibiotics, federal efforts to improve

antibiotics. They also include policies to reduce FDA approval times, thereby allowing manufacturers to obtain a return on their investments earlier, and tax breaks to defray the cost of the FDA approval process.

### :: REDUCING INCENTIVES TO OVERSELL EXISTING DRUGS

Even if pharmaceutical companies invest in developing new antibiotics, a significant problem remains: one firm's antibiotic sales generate cross-resistance to related antibiotics produced by other firms. The cross-resistance problem applies not just to antibiotics already on the market but also to those yet to be developed. Resistance generated by the use antibiotic management have been hindered by insufficient funding and attention. Since 1999, a U.S. Interagency Task Force on Antimicrobial Resistance, comprising representatives from the CDC, the FDA, the National Institutes of Health, and other agencies, has worked to bring greater attention to the resistance problem. Funding for the task force is lacking, however, and no lead agency is ultimately responsible for maintaining antibiotic effectiveness. Changing this would require congressional action recognizing a national interest in preserving antibiotic effectiveness and setting appropriations from the federal budget for a lead agency to coordinate the government's demand-side (antibiotic use) and supply-side (new antibiotic development) efforts. A congressional declaration that antibiotic effectiveness is a valuable societal resource could be a necessary step in resolving the "commons" problem inherent in antibiotic use, as it has for fisheries and waterways.

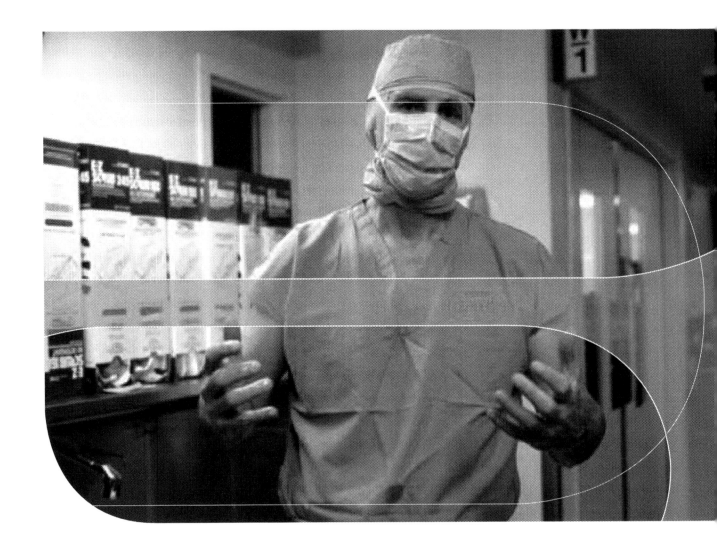

# Summary of Findings

1. **Antibiotic resistance is a threat to public health. Its root causes lie in insufficient incentives for patients, physicians, hospitals, and pharmaceutical companies to act in ways that would conserve antibiotic effectiveness.**

   - Antibiotic use by one patient eventually reduces drug effectiveness for everyone, but individual patients and physicians have little reason to consider this when deciding whether to take or prescribe an antibiotic.

   - Antibiotics are an inexpensive substitute for infection control. Hospitals have little incentive to fully consider the adverse impact of poor infection control practices because they share patients and problems with other facilities.

   - Even pharmaceutical companies, which have a profit motive to consider the effect of resistance on their antibiotics, are not motivated to think about resistance except as a market opportunity for new antibiotics. Several companies may have patents on different drugs that generate cross-resistance, so one pharmaceutical company has little incentive to care about resistance as long as other firms sell related drugs.

   - Research is needed to identify incentive-altering policies that could lower inappropriate antibiotic prescribing, encourage hospital infection control, and limit overselling and overusing antibiotics.

2. **Reducing inappropriate antibiotic use is important but potentially problematic from an incentives perspective because what is good for the patient conflicts with what is good for society.**

   - Appropriate antibiotic use not only benefits the patient but also limits spread of his infection to the community. Even incentives that specifically target inappropriate prescribing will encounter resistance, however, because they involve a tension between what is perceived to be good for the patient and what is good for society as a whole.

   - Discouraging inappropriate antibiotic use is widely acknowledged as a priority, but there is less agreement on exactly what kinds of prescribing are inappropriate and how they affect resistance. Current educational efforts should continue, but more research is needed on how to redesign physician incentives so that antibiotics are not used to substitute for time spent with the patient or other more time-intensive approaches.

   - Research should focus on identifying strategies to selectively reduce inappropriate prescribing.

3. **Demand-side solutions that do not put patients at risk are most feasible now.**

   - Expanding vaccination against pneumococcal bacteria either by mandate or through a subsidy would reduce the need for antibiotics. The vaccine is not used widely, however, because it is expensive and voluntary.

   - Development and deployment of a vaccine for MRSA may be a worthwhile public investment.

   - Subsidizing infection control in hospitals could encourage such practices as staff cohorting (assigning nursing staff to a small number of patients to prevent wider contact) and isolation of incoming patients colonized with resistant bacteria. Hospitals currently lack sufficient incentives to do this on their own, and regulations requiring hospitals to report levels of resistance and hospital infections can be circumvented.

4. **Encouraging research and development into new antibiotics may be effective at replenishing the pipeline of new antibiotics. But incentives for new drug development are incomplete solutions unless linked to greater incentives for pharmaceutical companies to care about resistance.**

   - Tax credits and other subsidies for new antibiotic development may help in the short term, but they do not solve the basic problem of cross-resistance among antibiotics that work in similar ways.

   - Efforts to protect new antibiotics from drug resistance

by keeping them on the sidelines potentially reduce incentives for new drug development by the pharmaceutical industry.

- Supply-side policies must encourage truly novel antibiotics—drugs that do not inherit the resistance problems created by their predecessors. Unless new antibiotics are developed, we will be confronted with the possibility of untreatable bacterial pathogens.

- Demand-side policies, such as reserving antibiotics for life-threatening situations, should take into account their effect on R&D investment for new antibiotics.

- Research should focus on grouping antibiotics by the extent to which they promote bacterial resistance to other antibiotics. These groupings are essential to defining adequate patent rights or the allowable scope of patent pools under antitrust law. They will also identify the truly novel antibiotics that perhaps ought to be subsidized. Research should also attempt to quantify the extent to which, for example, extending the Orphan Drug Act to new antibiotics might encourage investment in developing these drugs.

5. **Comprehensive antibiotic effectiveness legislation may be needed to protect a long-term sustainable future for antibiotic use.**

- Legislation recognizing the national interest in preserving antibiotic effectiveness would make the issue prominent. Explicitly recognizing the problem in the U.S. budget (with a budget line item, for example) and naming a lead agency would allow a coordinated government strategy to implement demand-side (antibiotic use) and supply-side (new antibiotic development) efforts.

- Congressional action to declare antibiotics a valuable societal resource may be helpful in resolving the commons problem inherent in antibiotic use, as it has been for fisheries.

- Policy research on natural resources legislation would assist in the design of comprehensive policies and legislation to extend antibiotic effectiveness.

# Next Steps:
## POLICY RESEARCH AND DIALOGUE

This report outlines various policy approaches to problems of antibiotic resistance, but assessing the approaches fully is challenged by gaps in the knowledge base. Our call for more data and research is not just a nod to the norm in such reports; we truly need more biological, medical, and economic analyses that can directly inform policy decisions. Although we have evaluated incentives and motivating factors from a theoretical perspective, policymakers will demand stronger evidence to act on policies like subsidizing infection control in hospitals. Pilot interventions are urgently needed, and the results of these experiments should be part of a national dialogue on what to do about antibiotic resistance.

At this time, death from drug-resistant pathogens, although increasing in frequency, is not yet a concern for most Americans. Many infections that are resistant to common antibiotics typically respond to other, more expensive drugs. However, running out of the cheapest antibiotics is somewhat like running out of oil. Just as oil is relatively cheap and convenient but not our only energy source, generic antibiotics are also inexpensive and available but may not be the only way to treat infectious diseases. Losing drugs that cost pennies a dose and moving to more expensive antibiotics, the newest of which can cost thousands of dollars per treatment, can have a profound impact on the health care system as a whole, and especially on the poor and uninsured, who are most likely to have to pay directly for their care.

Nevertheless, the time may come when even our most powerful antibiotics will fail. The proposals in this report are meant to offer a guide to policy and research to address this crisis now, rather than waiting until the pressure on policymakers to act—even in the absence of information—is unavoidable.

# References

**AHRQ (2003).** *Total Expenses for Conditions by Site of Service: United States, 2003: Medical Expenditure Panel Survey.* Rockville, MD: Agency for Health care Research and Quality.

**ASM (1994).** *Report of the ASM Task Force on Antibiotic Resistance.* http://www.asm.org/Policy/index.asp?bid=5961 (accessed May 31, 2006). American Society of Microbiology.

**Bell, J. M. and J. D. Turnidge. (2002).** "High Prevalence of Oxacillin-Resistant *Staphylococcus aureus* Isolates from Hospitalized Patients in Asia-Pacific and South Africa: Results from SENTRY Antimicrobial Surveillance Program, 1998-1999." *Antimicrobial Agents and Chemotherapy* 46(3): 879-881.

**Bosso, J. A. (2005).** "The Antimicrobial Armamentarium: Evaluating Current and Future Treatment Options." *Pharmacotherapy* 25(10 Pt 2): 55S-62S.

**CDC (1993).** "Nosocomial Enterococci Resistant to Vancomycin—United States, 1989-1993." *MMWR. Morbidity and Mortality Weekly Report* 42(30): 597-9. Centers for Disease Control and Prevention.

—— **(1999).** "National Nosocomial Infections Surveillance (NNIS) System Report, Data Summary from January 1990-May 1999, Issued June 1999." *American Journal of Infection Control* 27(6): 520-532.

—— **(2000).** "National Nosocomial Infections Surveillance (NNIS) System Report, Data Summary from January 1992-April 2000, Issued June 2000." *American Journal of Infection Control* 28(6): 429-448.

—— **(2001).** "National Nosocomial Infections Surveillance (NNIS) System Report, Data Summary from January 1992-June 2001, Issued August 2001." *American Journal of Infection Control* 29(6): 404-421.

—— **(2003).** "National Nosocomial Infections Surveillance (NNIS) System Report, Data Summary from January 1992 Through June 2003, Issued August 2003." *American Journal of Infection Control* 31(8): 481-498.

—— **(2004).** "National Nosocomial Infections Surveillance (NNIS) System Report, Data Summary from January 1992 Through June 2004, Issued October 2004." *American Journal of Infection Control* 32(8): 470-485.

—— **(2005).** Active Bacterial Core Surveillance Report: *Streptococcus pneumoniae*, 2005—Provisional. http://www.cdc.gov/ncidod/dbmd/abcs/survreports/spneu05prelim.pdf (accessed May 31, 2006).

**DeFrances C. J., M. J. Hall, et al. (2005).** "2003 National Hospital Discharge Survey. Advance Data from Vital and Health Statistics; No. 359." Hyattsville, MD: US Department of Health and Human Services, CDC, National Center for Health Statistics. http://www.cdc.gov/nchs/data/ad/ad359.pdf (accessed December 19, 2006).

**Diekema, D. J., M. A. Pfaller, et al. (2000).** "Trends in Antimicrobial Susceptibility of Bacterial Pathogens Isolated from Patients with Bloodstream Infections in the USA, Canada and Latin America." *International Journal of Antimicrobial Agents* 13(4): 257-271.

**Gerberding, J. (2003).** "The Centers for Disease Control and Prevention's Campaign to Prevent Antimicrobial Resistance in Health care Settings." *The Resistance Phenomenon in Microbes and Infectious Disease Vectors: Implications for Human Health and Strategies for Containment—Workshop Summary.* Knobler, S. L., S. M. Lemon, et al. (eds.). Washington, DC: National Academies Press, 210-215.

**Goossens, H., M. Ferech, et al. (2003).** "European Surveillance of Antibiotic Consumption (ESAC) Interactive Database." http://www.esac.ua.ac.be (accessed January 20, 2006).

**Hardin, G. (1968).** "The Tragedy of the Commons." *Science* 162: 1243-1248.

**Harrison, P. F. and J. Lederberg. (eds.) (1998).** *Antimicrobial Resistance: Issues and Options, Workshop Report.* Forum on Emerging Infections. Washington, DC: Institute of Medicine.

Howard, D. and K. Rask (2002). "The Impact of Resistance on Antibiotic Demand in Patients with Ear Infections." *Battling Resistance to Antibiotics and Pesticides: An Economic Approach.* R. Laxminarayan (ed.). Washington, DC: RFF Press: 119-133.

Interagency Task Force on Antimicrobial Resistance. (2001). *A Public Health Action Plan to Combat Antimicrobial Resistance, Part 1: Domestic Issues.* Washington, DC: U.S. Department of Health and Human Services.

Klein, E., D. L. Smith, and R. Laxminarayan. (2007). "Trends in Hospitalizations and Deaths in the United States Associated with Infections Caused by *Staphylococcus aureus* and MRSA, 1999–2004." Manuscript submitted for publication.

Laxminarayan, R. (2003). *Battling Resistance to Antibiotics and Pesticides: An Economic Approach.* Washington, DC: RFF Press.

Laxminarayan, R. and G. M. Brown. (2001). "Economics of Antibiotic Resistance: A Theory of Optimal Use." *Journal of Environmental Economics and Management* 42(2): 183-206.

Lee, K., Y. A. Kim, et al. (2004). "Increasing Prevalence of Vancomycin-Resistant Enterococci, and Cefoxitin-, Imipenem- and Fluoroquinolone-Resistant Gram-Negative Bacilli: A KONSAR Study in 2002." *Yonsei Medical Journal* 45(4): 598-608.

Lowy, F.D. (1998). "Staphylococcus aureus Infections." *The New England Journal of Medicine* 339(8): 520-532.

McDonald, L. C. (2006). "Trends in Antimicrobial Resistance in Health Care-Associated Pathogens and Effect on Treatment." *Clinical Infectious Diseases* 42(S2): S65-S71.

McManus, P., M. L. Hammond, et al. (1997). "Antibiotic Use in the Australian Community, 1990-1995." *The Medical Journal of Australia* 167(3): 124-7.

National Prescribing Service. (2005). "Antibiotic Prescribing Is Increasingly Judicious." *National Prescribing Service Newsletter* 40(June). http://www.nps.org.au/resources/NPS_News/news40/news40.pdf (accessed May 31, 2006).

OTA (1995). *Impact of Antibiotic-Resistant Bacteria: A Report to the U.S. Congress.* Office of Technology Assessment, Washington, DC: Government Printing Office.

RIVM (2005). "European Antimicrobial Resistance Surveillance System (EARSS)." http://www.rivm.nl/earss/ (accessed January 18, 2005), The National Institute for Public Health and the Environment.

Spellberg, B., J. H. Powers, et al. (2004). "Trends in Antimicrobial Drug Development: Implications for the Future." *Clinical Infectious Diseases* 38(9): 1279-86.

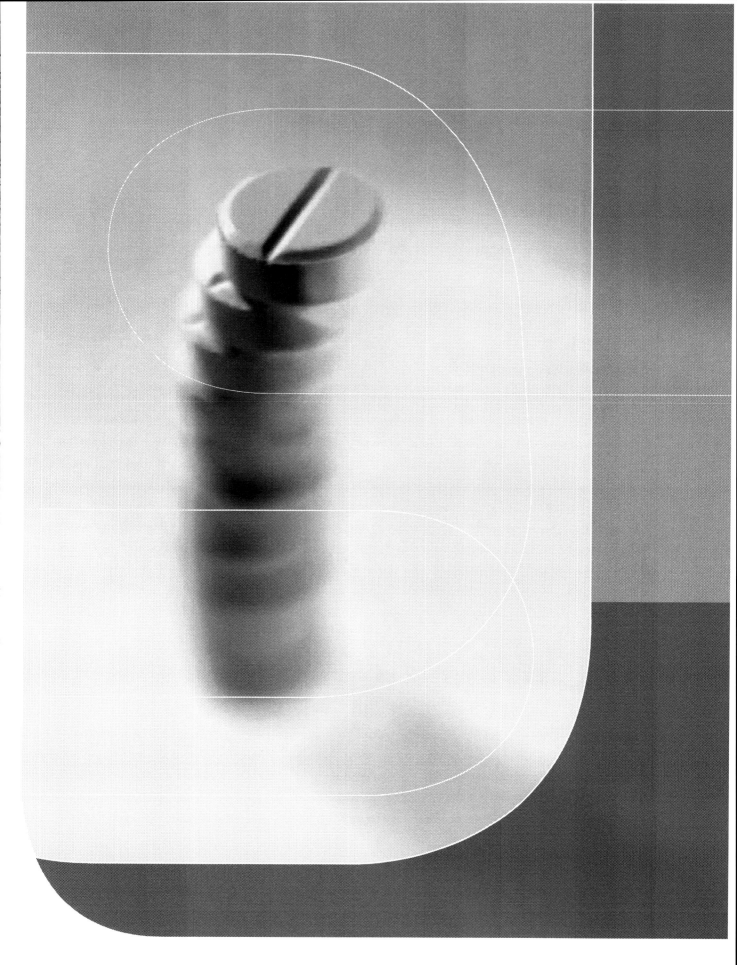

# Introduction

*Ramanan Laxminarayan*

From **The Lancet**, 1941

**Case 1.** *Policeman, aged 43.*

Admitted Oct. 12, 1940. Suppuration of face, scalp and both orbits, starting from a sore at the corner of the mouth a month earlier. Primary infection *Staph. aureus*; secondary, *Strep. pyogenes*. Sulphapyridine 19 g. given from Dec. 12 to 19; no improvement; drug-rash. Jan. 19: incision of multiple abscesses on face and scalp. ... [A] resulting arm-abscess, incised, gave *Staph. aureus* pus. General infection of left eye; cornea perforated Jan. 21. Eye eviscerated Feb. 3. Feb. 12: all incisions suppurating, in scalp, face, both orbits, and right arm. Lungs involved, with purulent expectoration containing both the pyogenic cocci. ... Penicillin 200 mg. given intravenously. ... Striking improvement after total of 800 mg. penicillin in 24 hours. Cessation of scalp discharge, diminution of right-eye suppuration and conjunctivitis. Arm discharge seemed less. ... Feb. 16: much improvement. ... Right eye almost normal. Some discharge still from left eye and arm. ... Feb. 17: penicillin supply exhausted. Total administered, 4.4 g. in 5 days. Patient felt much improved; no fever; appetite much better; resolution of infections in face, scalp and right orbit. —Abraham, Chain et al. 1941

From **The Washington Post**, January 27, 2006

Brandon Noble needs crutches to walk, and he has been relegated to spending much of his time at home on his sofa. When he's lying in bed at night and needs to move his left leg to get comfortable, he must lift it with his arms or nudge it with his right leg. He struggles to play with his children. But while Noble might have the typical limitations of a broken-down football player, the career of the Washington Redskins' defensive tackle isn't threatened by damaged ligaments or cracked bones. At 31, Noble has been sidelined by a staph infection, suffered after being injured, that in some cases is potentially fatal.

"It's been an incredible couple of years here," Noble said. "It's like I'm a modern-day Job." For the second time in a year, Noble is being treated for methicillin-resistant *Staphylococcus aureus*, or MRSA, a sometimes debilitating illness that is becoming increasingly common in the general population, according to national health experts. It is a growing concern for the NFL, which has experienced a recent increase in MRSA cases. —Maske and La Canfora 2006

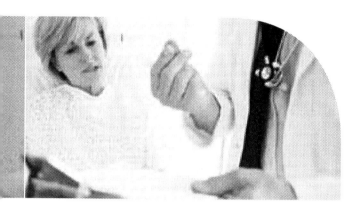

The excerpt from *The Lancet* describes the first-ever patient cured by penicillin—a policeman suffering from an invasive infection that had begun with a simple thorn scratch on his cheek. As difficult as it is to imagine today, our ability to treat common bacterial infections goes back only 65 years. Yet the rapid rate of emergence of pathogens resistant to these wonder drugs has already returned us to an era when community-acquired, difficult-to-treat strains of *Staphylococcus aureus* are increasingly common. A simple scratch can lead not just to painful death for sick patients in hospitals but to long, debilitating illnesses even for healthy athletes, as in the second excerpt, from *The Washington Post*.

Increasing bacterial resistance to antibiotics is a leading problem facing the public health community both in the United States and abroad. Pneumonia, sexually transmitted diseases, and infections of the skin and bowels are some of the illnesses that have become harder to treat because of drug resistance. An indication of the scale of the problem is given by the prevalence of high-level penicillin resistance in *Streptococcus pneumoniae* in the United States, which has risen from 0.02 percent in 1987 to over 20 percent in 2004 (CDC 2005). From 1974 to 2004, the prevalence of methicillin-resistant *Staphylococcus aureus* (MRSA) in hospitals has climbed from roughly 2 percent to more than 50 percent in many U.S. hospitals. According to the U.S. Food and Drug

Administration, "Unless antibiotic resistance problems are detected as they emerge, and actions are taken to contain them, the world could be faced with previously treatable diseases that have again become untreatable, as in the days before antibiotics were developed."

The impact of this long-heralded crisis is unfolding in hospitals and communities across the United States. According to the Centers for Disease Control and Prevention, 2 million patients in American hospitals each year are infected during their hospital stay. Of these, 90,000 die; in 70 percent of the cases, the bacteria that kill them are resistant to at least one commonly used antibiotic. This means that every day in the United States, approximately 172 men, women, and children—63,000 or more every year—die from infections caused by antibiotic-resistant bacteria in hospitals alone. The number, which exceeds U.S. mortality from AIDS, may actually be higher because many deaths attributed to other causes, particularly those of elderly patients suffering from a myriad of problems, may in reality be due to antibiotic-resistant infections.

Major reports in recent years have called for steps to address this growing threat before it engulfs the medical system (ASM 1994; OTA 1995; Harrison and Lederberg 1998), yet there has been astonishingly little action from policymakers. Antibiotics continue to be used widely both in medicine and in agriculture for growth promotion, and there are few requirements for hospitals to contain the spread of resistant pathogens. Confusion over antibiotic resistance in the public policy realm arises, in part, because the medical community is grappling with what is essentially a problem of missing incentives. Those who use antibiotics, be they patients, physicians, or farmers, have few incentives to consider the negative impact of that use on society. In the language of economists, antibiotic resistance is a negative "externality" associated with the use of antibiotics, much as pollution is an undesirable externality associated with the use of automobiles. Standard responses like increasing surveillance and launching public information campaigns on the hazards of resistance—however necessary a part of an overall policy response—may have only a limited impact. Moreover, the problem of antibiotic resistance is not restricted to how antibiotics are used but is related to other factors, such as infection control and patent law. Viewed broadly, antibiotic resistance is both a biological and a behavioral problem that needs a combination of technological, educational, and incentive-based responses.

In this report, we examine the problem of antibiotic resistance from a natural resources and incentive-based perspective. We explore policy solutions that will enable society to make the best use of existing antibiotics, sensibly encourage the discovery of new antibiotics, and give drug firms a greater incentive to sell these new drugs responsibly. We describe specific actions and changes that, if implemented, could have a lasting impact on our ability to use antibiotics in a sustainable manner. The proposed changes go beyond simply tinkering with the current system; we identify deep weaknesses in how we develop, regulate, and use antibiotics.

This report is the result of a two-year study by researchers at Resources for the Future, the University of Chicago, the National Institutes of Health, and Emory University. It objectively evaluates a range of policy options for dealing with antibiotic resistance. The policy options discussed in this report were debated at four consultations with clinicians, epidemiologists, lawyers, economists, and representatives from hospitals, health insurance and managed-care organizations, health care quality organizations, accreditation agencies, pharmaceutical companies, and government agencies; participants provided invaluable insights into the incentives behind choices concerning antibiotic use and development. Each consultation dealt with a specific set of issues: supply of new antibiotics, payers' incentives with respect to resistance, role for government agencies, and incentives for health care providers. Our purpose at this stage was not to try to develop consensus around any specific policy proposal, but rather to have each policy idea evaluated as critically as current evidence would permit and to identify knowledge gaps that prevented a more informed evaluation. The study focused on antibiotic use in medicine and did not explicitly address the problem of antibiotic overuse in agriculture for growth promotion, but clearly it is also important to change incentives for how the drugs are used in that context.

The next phase of the Extending the Cure project will expand the process of policy research and dialogue and develop a comprehensive manual of incentive-based policy options that government and other policymakers can use to make a real difference in the fight against antibiotic resistance.

■

## Antibiotic effectiveness as a natural resource

Antibiotic effectiveness is a natural resource, much like oil, fish, or trees. Whether effectiveness is renewable (like trees or fish) or nonrenewable (like oil) depends on whether resistance declines when antibiotic use is withdrawn.[1] Any antibiotic use today, whether appropriate or not, imposes selection pressure on resistant bacteria that diminishes our ability to use the antibiotic in the future. The fundamental tension between how we use antibiotics today and our ability to use them in the future offers crucial insights for thinking about drug resistance (Laxminarayan and Brown 2001; Laxminarayan 2003).

Just as it is difficult to create a policy to manage a cod fishery optimally without understanding the biological dynamics of fish, an effort to craft policy solutions to the antibiotic resistance problem requires a clear understanding of the evolutionary biology of resistance. The problem of resistance

---

1   This is determined by the fitness cost of resistance—the evolutionary disadvantage of resistant strains in the absence of antibiotics. See Chapter 2 for a more complete discussion.

is, at its heart, an evolutionary game played between humans and microbes: humans try to stay ahead of microbes by creating new antibiotics, and microbes evolve by developing resistance to our drugs. Unfortunately for humans, microbes evolve resistance to antibiotics faster than we are likely to create new ones. The basic evolutionary biology and epidemiology of resistance and their relationship to potential policy levers are described in Chapter 2 of this report.

Antibiotics are different from other resources in that their use has both positive and negative externalities (impacts on other people). The negative impact is that, just as one fisherman's catch makes other fishermen worse off by leaving fewer fish in the ocean, one patient's use of antibiotics makes other people worse off by increasing the likelihood that their infection may not be treatable. The positive impact, however, is that the patient's use of antibiotic could make other people *better* off by reducing the risk that his infection will be passed on to them.

Dealing with antibiotic resistance does not always place individual well-being at odds with that of the rest of society. An effective way of lowering the need for antibiotics is preventing the spread of infection through better infection control in hospitals and other health care settings and in the community, particularly in places like day-care centers and nursing homes. Vaccination also has the potential to lower the need for antibiotics (a vaccine to prevent pneumococcal disease is already available). However, as long as antibiotics are inexpensive to the patient—because of low-cost generics or insurance coverage or both—they are used as a substitute for other forms of infection control.

Antibiotic effectiveness is an open-access resource that any individual physician or patient can tap. Even a pharmaceutical firm that owns a patent on an antibiotic does not control its effectiveness, since other firms likely manufacture similar

## Antibiotic effectiveness is an open-access resource that any individual physician or patient can tap.

drugs in the same class of antibiotics.[2] An important condition for the wise use of a natural resource is that there be clear and well-defined ownership. When there is no clear owner, then many users acting in their own self-interest tend to overuse the resource, leading to collapse, as famously described by Garrett Hardin in his paper, "The Tragedy of the Commons" (1968).[3] Private ownership offers individual owners an incentive to conserve a resource so as not to diminish its future value (Scott 1955; Buchanan 1956). Since there is no single owner of antibiotic effectiveness in any single "functional resistance group"[4] of antibiotics, suboptimal use is unavoidable. The incentives that shape the behavior of patients, physicians, and health care organizations, including hospitals, when dealing with drug resistance are addressed in Chapters 3 and 4.

The potential for overuse and misuse of antibiotics leads to market failures that justify regulatory intervention. Antibiotics are fundamentally different from other drugs because of the resistance externality, but for the most part, the system by which they are approved and used fails to recognize their special status. The government may have a

---

2  Bacteria resistant to a specific antibiotic may also be protected from similar antibiotics without the need for any additional mutation.

3  The important caveat, as described by Anthony Scott, is that "the property must be allocated on a *scale* sufficient to insure that one management has complete control of the asset" (Scott 1955).

4  We use the term *functional resistance group* in a way distinct from the more common use of antibiotic classes. Today there are 16 classes of antibiotics, but there is often cross-resistance between different classes. Use of an antibiotic affects resistance to other drugs within the same resistance class but not to drugs in other resistance classes. See Box 2.1 (in Chapter 2) for a more complete explanation.

role to play in ensuring that antibiotic effectiveness is used carefully. The roles of other federal agencies, like the Centers for Disease Control and Prevention (CDC), the Food and Drug Administration (FDA), and the National Institutes of Health (NIH), are addressed in Chapter 5, and the specific role of Medicare and Medicaid is discussed in Chapter 6.

Finally, we can draw important lessons in how to stimulate research and development into new antibiotics by studying other natural resources and understanding the tension between making better use of antibiotics and investing in new antibiotics (Chapter 7). In the past few decades we have become familiar with the tension between making better use of existing oil resources and exploration for new oil fields. Improving the efficiency with which we use oil lowers the incentives to invest in exploration, and conversely, an increase in exploration activity can lower the value of current stocks of oil. Similarly, efforts to make better use of existing antibiotics by discouraging inappropriate prescribing by physicians or misuse by patients can help slow the development of resistance but also reduce incentives for pharmaceutical manufacturers to invest in new antibiotics. And efforts to restrict antibiotic use or to conserve new, powerful antibiotics for emergency situations also have consequences for incentives to develop new antibiotics.

The insights that emerge from thinking about antibiotic effectiveness as a societal resource are useful as we search for policy solutions. However, these broad insights, without greater detail, can get lost in the context of the complex, largely privately financed U.S. health care system. Therefore, we begin from a natural resources approach but go beyond this analogy to examine potential responses to the resistance challenge within the details, realities, and constraints of health care practice in the United States. The authors of this report discuss policy recommendations and offer open questions and researchable topics that will be critical for shaping policy solutions.

At this time, death from a drug-resistant pathogen, although increasing in frequency, is not yet a concern for most Americans. Many infections that are resistant to common antibiotics typically respond to other, more expensive drugs. However, running out of the cheapest antibiotics is somewhat like running out of oil. Just as oil is relatively cheap and convenient but not our only energy source, so generic antibiotics are inexpensive and available but may not be the only way to treat infectious diseases. Losing drugs that cost pennies a dose and moving to more expensive antibiotics, the newest of which can cost thousands of dollars, can have a profound impact on the health care system as a whole, and especially on the poor and uninsured, who are most likely to have to pay for some part of their care.

Nevertheless, there may come a time when even our more powerful antibiotics will no longer be consistently effective against certain types of bacteria. The proposals in this report are meant to offer a guide to prepare for and respond to the inevitable crisis, when there will undoubtedly be far greater pressure on policymakers to act.[5]

---

5    Sadly, most policy responses tend to come *ex post* rather than in preparation for a crisis. For example, in 1937, while Congress debated the regulation of pharmaceuticals, 107 people, mostly children, died from Elixir Sulfanilamide, which contained the poisonous solvent diethylene glycol. That incident prompted passage of the Federal Food, Drug, and Cosmetic Act of 1938, which required that the safety of new drugs be demonstrated before they could be marketed and sold.

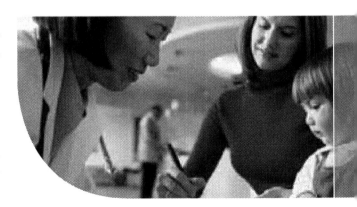

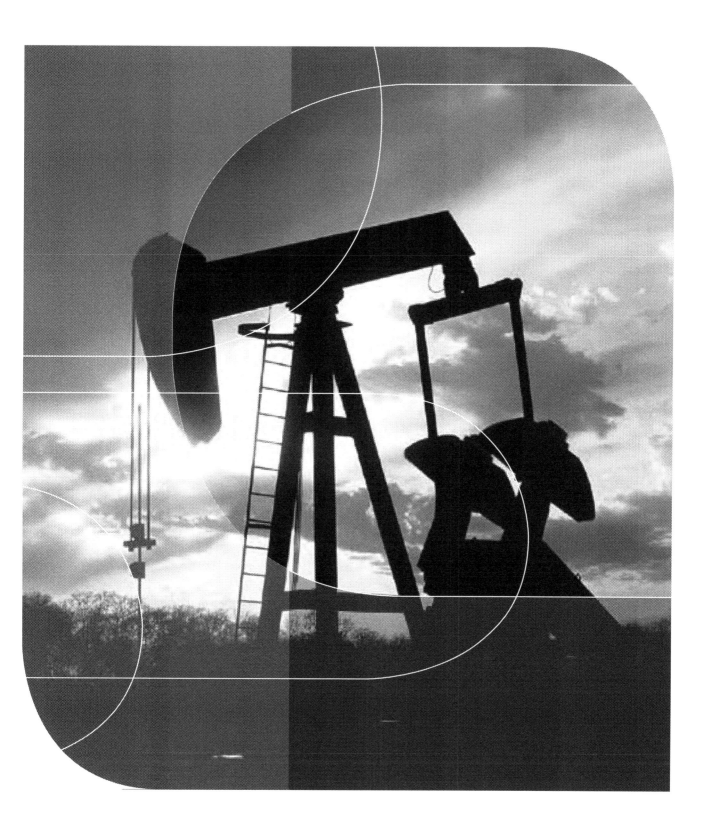

# References

**Abraham, E. P., E. Chain, et al. (1941).** "Further Observations on Penicillin." *The Lancet* 231(6155): 177-89.

**ASM (1994).** *Report of the ASM Task Force on Antibiotic Resistance.* http://www.asm.org/Policy/index.asp?bid=5961 (accessed May 31, 2006). American Society of Microbiology.

**Buchanan, J. M. (1956).** "Private Ownership and Common Usage: The Road Case Reexamined." *Southern Economic Journal* 22: 305-16.

**CDC (2005).** *Active Bacterial Core Surveillance Report*: Streptococcus pneumoniae, *2005—Provisional.* http://www.cdc.gov/ncidod/dbmd/abcs/survreports/spneu05prelim.pdf (accessed May 31, 2006). Centers for Disease Control and Prevention.

**Hardin, G. (1968).** "The Tragedy of the Commons." *Science* 162: 1243-1248.

**Harrison, P. F. and J. Lederberg (eds.). (1998).** *Antimicrobial Resistance: Issues and Options, Workshop report.* Forum on Emerging Infections. Washington, DC: Institute of Medicine.

**Maske, M. and J. La Canfora. (2006).** "A Frightening Off-Field Foe: Redskins' Noble Battles Infection That Is Growing Concern for NFL" *The Washington Post,* Jan. 27, E1.

**Laxminarayan, R. (2003).** *Battling Resistance to Antibiotics and Pesticides: An Economic Approach.* Washington, DC: RFF Press.

**Laxminarayan, R. and G. M. Brown. (2001).** "Economics of Antibiotic Resistance: A Theory of Optimal Use." *Journal of Environmental Economics and Management* 42(2): 183-206.

**OTA (1995).** *Impacts of Antibiotic-Resistant Bacteria: A Report to the U.S. Congress.* OTA-H-629. Washington, DC: Government Printing Office. Office of Technology Assessment.

**Scott, A. (1955).** "The Fishery: The Objectives of Sole Ownership." *Journal of Political Economy* 63: 116-124.

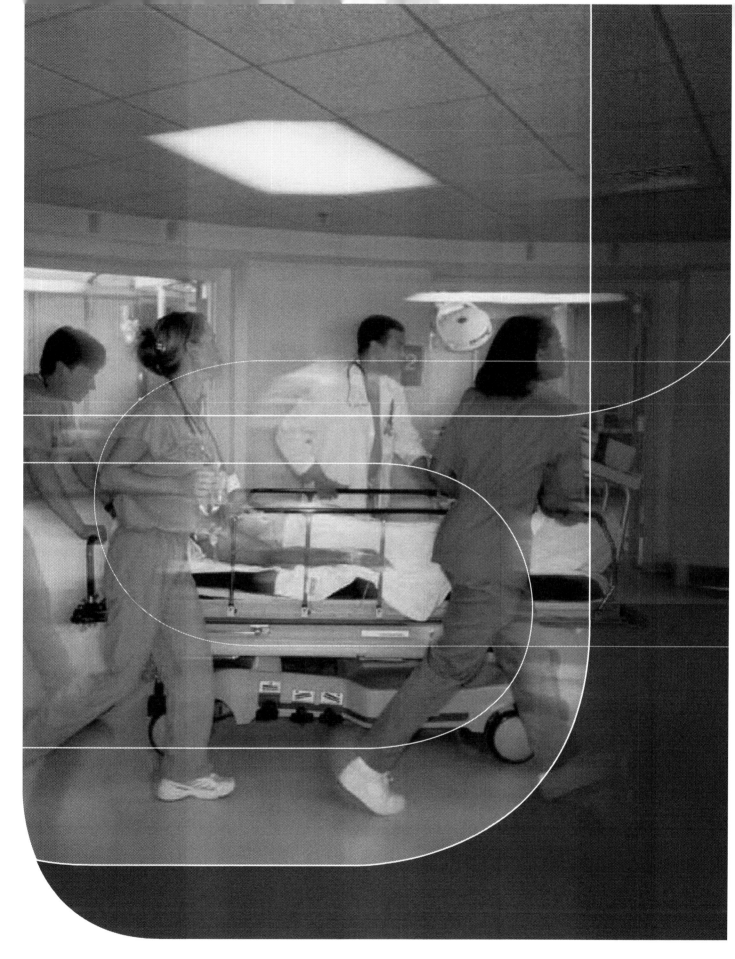

# Antibiotic resistance: **The unfolding crisis**

*Ramanan Laxminarayan*

The introduction of penicillin in 1941 is among the most significant technological advances in modern medicine. Although many improvements in public health and medicine and a decline in infectious disease mortality preceded the introduction of penicillin, antibiotics have made possible further reductions in deaths and disability from infectious disease (Figure 1.1). Perhaps equally important, they have facilitated the vast expansion of other medical interventions, such as kidney and heart transplants, by allowing clinicians to prevent surgical site infections and infections in immuno-suppressed patients, such as organ recipients. Now, growing levels of bacterial resistance to antibiotics threaten our ability not just to treat infectious diseases but also to perform other procedures and treatments that fundamentally depend on affordable and effective antibiotics.

The timeline of emergence of drug resistance is best illustrated by the case of *Staphylococcus aureus (S. aureus)*, a common pathogen that causes life-threatening infections and is transmitted in both health care and community settings. The mortality rate from a *S. aureus* infection was as high as 82 percent in the preantibiotics era (Skinner and Keefer 1941) but fell dramatically after the introduction of penicillin. Resistance to penicillin emerged soon after its introduction

and was linked to patient deaths in the early 1950s (Abboud and Waisbren 1959). In 1960, penicillin was replaced with a beta-lactam compound, methicillin, which was effective against penicillin-resistant *S. aureus*, but methicillin-resistant *S. aureus* (MRSA) emerged in the 1970s in Europe and soon after in the United States. MRSA prevalence in U.S. hospitals, which was 2.4 percent in 1975, increased to 29 percent in 1991 (Archer 1998) (Figure 1.2), and 59.5 percent in 2003

FIGURE 1.1

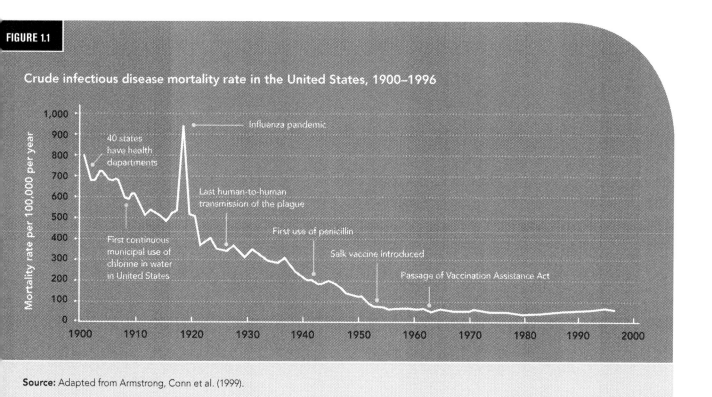

Crude infectious disease mortality rate in the United States, 1900–1996

**Source:** Adapted from Armstrong, Conn et al. (1999).

(CDC 2004), growing at an average rate of more than 12 percent per year. Vancomycin is the main and potentially last available drug that can reliably treat MRSA infections, and the massive use of vancomycin for treating MRSA is believed to be an important reason for the emergence and spread of vancomycin-resistant enterococci (VRE) (Weinstein 2003). Meanwhile, strains of MRSA resistant to vancomycin have been detected, providing the first glimpse of medical outcomes in a post-antibiotics era (Chang, Sievert et al. 2003).

The fast evolution of *S. aureus* from a bacterium that was easily treatable at pennies a dose to a pathogen that now requires powerful, expensive antibiotics is paralleled by other predominantly hospital-acquired infections, like those caused by VRE, Enterobacter and *Pseudomonas aeruginosa*. In each case, the ability to treat bacterial infections has been rolled back by the evolution of resistance. In this chapter, we describe the medical and economic impacts of resistance and explore why drug resistance is a compelling problem that, if left unaddressed, has the potential to derail the health care system by returning us to a world where children, the elderly, and other vulnerable populations routinely die from simple bacterial infections.

### Trends in resistance

The pathogens that are transmitted in hospitals and communities are different in their ecology and epidemiology, as explained in Chapter 2. Drug resistance is growing in both types of pathogens. Common hospital-acquired, or nosocomial, infections include Gram-positive infections, such as those caused by *S. aureus* and enterococci, whose resistance has been increasing at a rapid pace. In 1998, MRSA was detected among patients without recent health care exposure or other predisposing risk factors (Herold, Immergluck et al. 1998), and it has since become an important threat to community health.

Resistance has become a serious problem among hospital-acquired Gram-negative pathogens, such as *Escherichia coli*, *Acinetobacter baumannii*, *Klebsiella pneumoniae,* and *Pseudomonas aeruginosa*, as shown in Figure 1.3 (Gaynes and Edwards 2005). Gram-negative pathogens are even more challenging than MRSA because there are fewer antibiotics available to treat infections caused by them.

■

## Comparison with other countries

Hospitals in the United States have among the highest rates of MRSA in the world: on average 60 percent of patients infected with *S. aureus* in intensive care units of U.S. hospitals cannot be treated with methicillin or older antibiotics (CDC 2004). Surveillance for drug-resistant hospital-acquired infections has been less successful than in Europe, where a concerted effort has been made to identify antimicrobial rates in both hospital and community settings. Figure 1.4 shows MRSA rates for the United States and other high- and middle-income countries for 2004. In Europe, only Romania and Malta had higher rates of MRSA than the United States in that year. MRSA levels were high in East Asia, specifically South Korea, Japan, and Taiwan, probably because of high levels of antibiotic use, but not much higher than for the United States. In the Americas, only Argentina, Brazil, and Colombia had a higher MRSA prevalence than the United States.

Prevalence of vancomycin-resistant enterococci (VRE) in U.S. hospitals is estimated to be roughly 12 percent on average across all hospital patients (McDonald 2006) and according to the CDC is more than 28 percent in intensive care units

(CDC 2004). VRE rates in the United States and other countries are shown in Figure 1.5. In Europe, only Portugal had a higher prevalence of VRE than did the United States. Data on VRE prevalence outside Europe are less reliable but show lower rates than the United States, with the exception of South Korea. Reliable studies from Japan have found isolated outbreaks but no evidence of VRE transmission (Arakawa, Ike et al. 2000; Matsumoto, Muratani et al. 2004).

One reason for the higher prevalence of resistance in the United States may be the higher levels of antibiotic

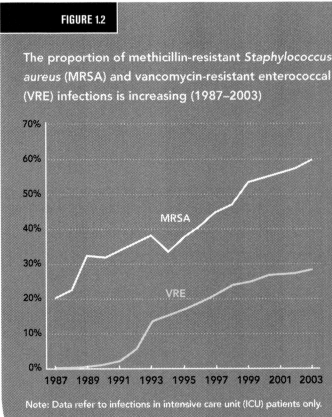

### FIGURE 1.2

The proportion of methicillin-resistant *Staphylococcus aureus* (MRSA) and vancomycin-resistant enterococcal (VRE) infections is increasing (1987–2003)

Note: Data refer to infections in intensive care unit (ICU) patients only.

**Sources:** VRE and MRSA data, 1998–2000, 2002–2003 (CDC 1999; CDC 2000; CDC 2001; CDC 2003; CDC 2004); data for 2001 are the average of 2000 and 2002 data. MRSA data from 1987–1997 are estimated from (Lowy 1998). VRE data for 1989 and 1993 are from (CDC 1993). VRE data for 1990–1992 and 1994–1997 are interpolated based on geometric mean.

FIGURE 1.3

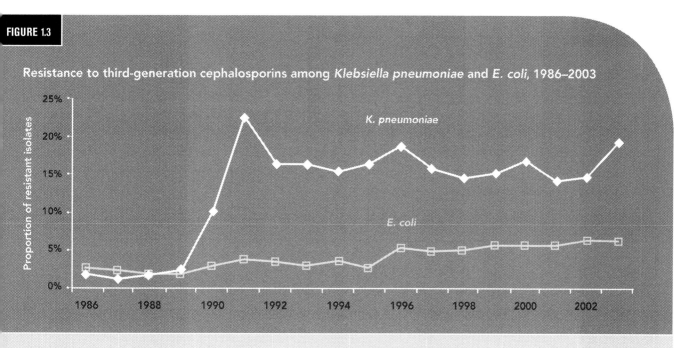

**Resistance to third-generation cephalosporins among *Klebsiella pneumoniae* and *E. coli*, 1986–2003**

**Source:** Adapted from Gaynes and Edwards (2005).

prescribing in this country (see Box 2.5, Chapter 2). Although antibiotic prescribing has fallen in the United States since 1994, it remains among the highest in the world (Steinman, Gonzales et al. 2003). Data from the European Surveillance of Antibiotic Consumption (Goossens, Ferech et al. 2003) show prescribing rates for most countries from 1997 to 2002 (Figure 1.6). The prescribing rate in the United States was 24 defined daily doses per 1,000 population per year. Only five countries—France, Luxembourg, Italy, Greece, and Portugal—had higher rates, but some of these countries had lower rates of resistance than the United States, indicating that there may be other casual factors.

### Health impact of drug resistance

Patients who have a hospital infection have a lower probability of survival (Osmon, Warren et al. 2003), as shown in Figure 1.7. This survival disadvantage is worse if the infection is due to a drug-resistant pathogen. Studies have shown that patients infected with resistant strains of bacteria are more likely to require longer hospitalization (Holmberg, Solomon et al. 1987; The Genesis Report 1994) and are more likely to die. For instance, the mortality rate for patients infected with MRSA has been found to be significantly higher than for patients infected with a methicillin-sensitive strain (Rubin, Harrington et al. 1999; Blot et al. 2002; Cosgrove et al. 2005).

Estimating the number of people who die from drug-resistant infections is challenging, for a number of reasons. First, patients who get resistant infections tend to be older and sicker, and therefore it is difficult to separate the impact of having a resistant infection from other complications they may have, such as HIV or TB co-infection (in community settings). Second, drug-resistant infections are not coded differently from sensitive infections. Therefore, most estimates

## WHY MULTIPLE ANTIBIOTICS USED IN COMBINATION MINIMIZE RISK OF TREATMENT FAILURE

Let us assume that with probability $q$, a doctor finds acceptable as a threshold probability that at least one of the antibiotics used to treat the patient will work. Suppose there are $n$ antibiotics. The probability that the infection is treated by any single antibiotic is $p$, the probability that the drug will not work is $(1-p)$, and the probability that none of the drugs will work is $(1-p)^n$. Consequently, the rule to choose $n$, the number of antibiotics so that the patient will recover without needing a second course of medications, is

$$1-(1-p)^n > q$$

If $q = .95$ and $p = 0.7$, then we can easily calculate that $n$ must be at least 3. Even if each drug is 70 percent effective, the patient must be prescribed three antibiotics in combination to ensure that there is a less than 5 percent chance of treatment failure.

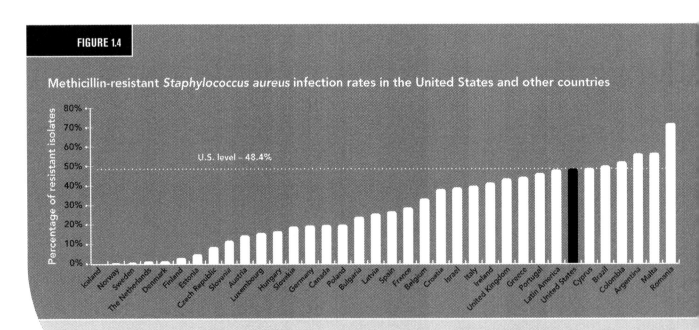

Methicillin-resistant *Staphylococcus aureus* infection rates in the United States and other countries

**Sources:** Canada and United States, 2000–2002 (Jones, Draghi et al. 2004); Latin America, 1998 (Diekema, Pfaller et al. 2000); Brazil, 1998 (Melo, Silva-Carvalho et al. 2004); Colombia, 2001–2002 (Arias, Reyes et al. 2003); Argentina, 2002 (Bantar, Famiglietti et al. 2004); European countries, 2004 (RIVM 2005).

FIGURE 1.5

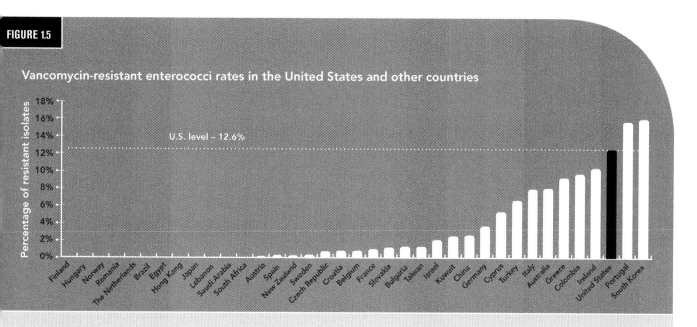

Vancomycin-resistant enterococci rates in the United States and other countries

U.S. level – 12.6%

**Sources:** Brazil, 2002 (Titze-de-Almeida, Filho et al. 2004); Egypt, Lebanon, Saudi Arabia, South Africa, and Turkey, 2001–2002 (Bouchillon, Johnson et al. 2004); Hong Kong, 2000 (Ho 2003); Japan, 2000 (Arakawa, Ike et al. 2000); New Zealand, 2000 (Briggs, Upton et al. 2002); Taiwan and United States, 2000 (McDonald, Lauderdale et al. 2004); Kuwait, 1999–2001 (Udo, Al-Sweih et al. 2003); Australia, 1999 (Nimmo, Bell et al. 2003); Colombia, 2001–2002 (Arias, Reyes et al. 2003); China (Liu, Xu et al. 2003); South Korea, 2002 (Lee, Kim et al. 2004); European countries, 2004 (RIVM 2005).

of the burden of drug resistance are based on the number of infections multiplied by resistance percentages. One such study that used data from the National Hospital Discharge Survey (NHDS) found 125,969 hospitalizations for MRSA between 1999 and 2000. These accounted for 3.95 of more than 1,000 hospitalizations (compared with a diagnosis of *S. aureus* infection in 9.13 of every 1,000 hospitalizations) (Kuehnert, Hill et al. 2005). Estimates of methicillin resistance in this study indicated that older patients were most likely to have an MRSA infection (6.36 per 1,000 hospitalizations for those above age 65, compared with 1.31 per 1,000 hospitalizations for those aged 14 and under). A 1995 CDC study, unpublished but cited in Kuehnert, Hill et al. (2005) and based on data from NHDS and the National Nosocomial Infections Surveillance System (NNIS), found that *S. aureus* infections accounted for 0.58 percent of hospitalizations and MRSA accounted for 0.2 percent of hospitalizations.

Estimates based on more recent data are presented in Table 1.1 of this report.

## Economic impact of resistance

Drug resistance places a burden on patients, hospitals, and the health care system. The annual figures quoted most often for the economic impact of resistance in the United States range from $350 million to $35 billion (in 1989 dollars). These estimates assume that 150 million prescriptions are generated each year and vary with, among other factors, the rate at which resistance grows with respect to increasing antibiotic use, and the probability that a patient will die following infection with a resistant pathogen (Phelps 1989). A recent study that measures the deadweight loss from antibiotic resistance associated with outpatient prescriptions in the

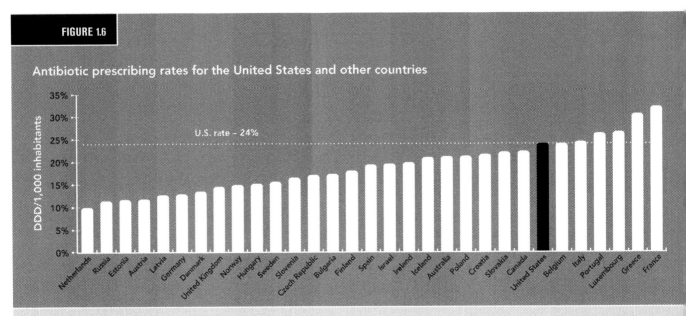

**FIGURE 1.6**

Antibiotic prescribing rates for the United States and other countries

U.S. rate – 24%

DDD/1,000 inhabitants

Netherlands, Russia, Estonia, Austria, Latvia, Germany, Denmark, United Kingdom, Norway, Hungary, Sweden, Slovenia, Czech Republic, Bulgaria, Finland, Spain, Israel, Ireland, Iceland, Australia, Poland, Croatia, Slovakia, Canada, United States, Belgium, Italy, Portugal, Luxembourg, Greece, France

**Sources:** Canada, Australia, and United States, 1994 (McManus, Hammond et al. 1997); Russia, 1998 (Cizman, Beovic et al. 2004); Australia, 2002 (National Prescribing Service 2005); European countries, 2004 (Goossens, Ferech et al. 2003).
**Note:** DDD=defined daily doses, a standardized measure of antibiotic consumption.

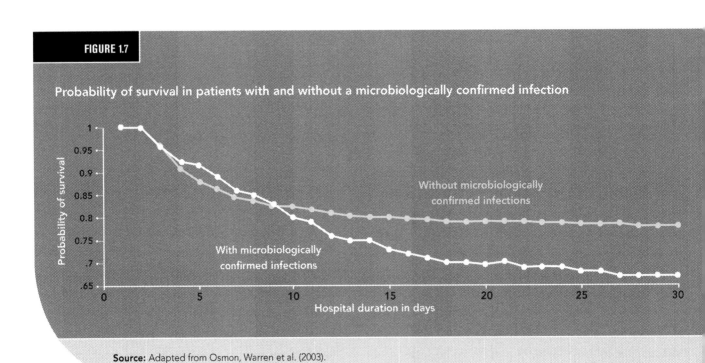

**FIGURE 1.7**

Probability of survival in patients with and without a microbiologically confirmed infection

Without microbiologically confirmed infections

With microbiologically confirmed infections

Probability of survival

Hospital duration in days

**Source:** Adapted from Osmon, Warren et al. (2003).

FIGURE 1.8

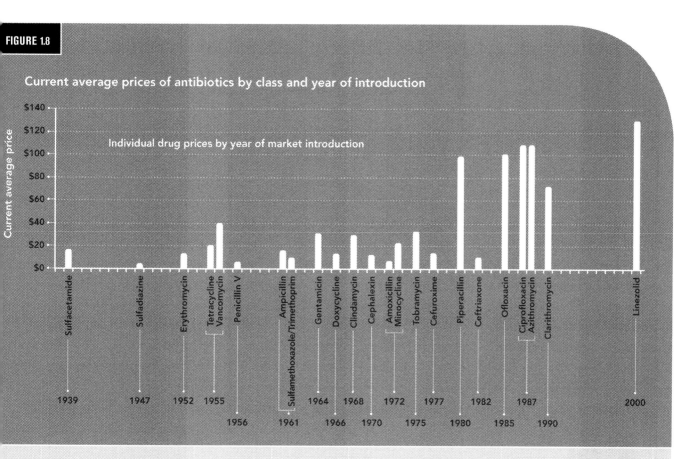

Current average prices of antibiotics by class and year of introduction

Note: Price data are the average of Federal Supply Schedule prices for individual drugs, which come from the Department of Veteran's Affairs. The individual drugs were grouped into the categories shown above according to the US Pharmacopeia Model Guidelines Drug List. The majority of prices are for 250mg dosage with the following exceptions: sulfamethoxazole/trimethoprim (800mg), piperacillin (various injections), gentamicin (various injections/solution), tobramycin (various injections/solution), sulfadiazine (1% cream), sulfacetamide (wash/lotion), doxycycline (100mg), minocycline (199mg), vancomycin (various injections), linezolid (100mg, 200mg), and clindamycin (300mg).

United States puts the cost at a minimum of $378 million and as high as $18.6 billion (Elbasha 2003). A report by the Office of Technology Assessment to the U.S. Congress estimated the annual cost associated with antibiotic resistance in hospitals, attributable to five classes of hospital-acquired infections from six species of antibiotic-resistant bacteria, to be at least $1.3 billion (in 1992 dollars) (OTA 1995). The CDC estimated that the cost of all hospital-acquired infections, including both antibiotic-resistant and antibiotic-susceptible strains, was $4.5 billion. The lack of time-series data on both antimicrobial use

and bacterial resistance has made it difficult to estimate the dose-response relationship between antimicrobial use and resistance. As a result, assessing resistance-related economic costs becomes more complicated. Although burden estimates can convey an idea of the overall size of the problem, they are usefully complemented by assessments of the economic benefit of lowering resistance—by, say, 10 percent—to evaluate the benefit-cost ratio of any particular policy.

Infections caused by antimicrobial-resistant bacteria result in increased morbidity and mortality for those affected and drive up health care costs as well. The costs and consequences associated with failing to address antimicrobial resistance arise on many levels. There is lost time at work and school, plus longer and repeated hospital stays. Given the variety of ways in which antibiotic resistance can impose direct and indirect costs, it should be no surprise that its financial burden is staggering. In fact, the Institute of Medicine estimates that the price tag may be as high as $30 billion a year (Palumbi 2001).

An analysis of U.S. inpatient hospital days in 2000 and 2001 found that 1 percent of all admissions acquire *S. aureus* infections, for a total of 300,000 cases and 2.7 million excess patient days per year (Noskin, Rubin et al. 2005). The study also found that length of stay for infected patients increased from 4.5 days to 14.3 days, there were 12,000 deaths, a 4 percent increase in in-hospital mortality, and the cost was estimated to be $9.5 billion a year. Another study that examined the economic impact of *S. aureus* in Canadian hospitals showed that MRSA infections resulted in, on average, 14 additional hospital days. In the same study, the total attributable cost to treat MRSA infections was

$14,360 per patient, and the cost for isolation and management of colonized patients was $1,363 per admission (Kim, Oh et al. 2001). A more complete description of the higher economic costs imposed by hospital-acquired drug-resistant infections is presented in Chapter 4.

Another significant burden imposed by drug resistance comes in the cost of periodic switches to newer, more expensive antibiotics. As the risk of treatment failure increases with resistance, the entire system has to shift over to new drugs even if older drugs retain substantial effectiveness. The increase in cost with successive generations has been enormous. Penicillin costs pennies a dose; the most recent antibiotics can run as high as a few thousand dollars for a course of treatment. (Newer antibiotics are more expensive largely because they are still on patent, and these costs will go down as they come off patent.) From the perspective of the health care system, these periodic upgrades to the antibiotics used most often for treatment impose a significant burden. The cost of patented drugs reflects monopoly rents to some extent, but also the significant and

---

**TABLE 1.1**

### ESTIMATED HOSPITAL-ACQUIRED INFECTIONS CAUSED BY METHICILLIN-RESISTANT *S. AUREUS* AND VANCOMYCIN-RESISTANT ENTEROCOCCI, 1995–2004

| RESISTANT BACTERIA | 1995 | 2000 | 2004 |
| --- | --- | --- | --- |
| Methicillin-resistant *S. aureus* | 70,000[†] | 125,969[‡] | 250,438[§] |
| Vancomycin-resistant enterococci | 14,000[†] | 20,710[*] | 26,085[*] |

**Sources:** ‡Kuehnert, Hill et al. 2005. *Klein, Laxminarayan 2006. †GAO 1999. §Klein, Smith et al. 2007.

real resource costs of investing in new antibiotics. Moreover, even with modest levels of resistance to antibiotics, patients have to be treated empirically with two or more drugs to ensure that treatment will be successful (Box 1.1). Sequential treatment with different antibiotics until the clinician hits upon one that works is not an option when patients are immuno-compromised and treatment failure could put their lives in jeopardy.

Figure 1.8 compares current (nominal) prices of different generations of antibiotics. There is a general increasing trend in prices, with newer antibiotics, such as oxazolidinones and quinolones, costing much more than penicillins, sulfonamides, and other older drugs. Since most antibiotics, with the exception of the most recent ones, are off patent, the higher cost of relatively newer drugs likely reflects the enormous regulatory costs of bringing a drug to market. To date, there has been only one analysis of the drug-related cost of bacterial resistance. Howard and Rask (2002) take 1980–1998 data on antibiotics used to treat ear infections from the National Ambulatory Medical Care Survey to estimate the increase in the cost of antibiotic treatment attributable to increases in bacterial resistance. Lacking data on resistance, they used time trends as a proxy for resistance to show that between 1997 and 1998, increases in drug resistance are estimated to have raised the cost of treating ear infections by about 20 percent ($216 million). This approach is not perfect, however, since time trends may capture costs unrelated to resistance, such as the costs of antibiotics with lower side-effect profiles or more convenient dosing.

■

## Discussion

Drug-resistant infections impose a significant cost on patients, health care systems, and society by increasing the cost of treating infections and causing greater disability and death. However, their impact is not restricted to infectious diseases. Many aspects of modern medicine—whether organ

transplants, chemotherapy, or surgery—require effective drugs that can ward off infection. In that sense, antibiotics can be considered a complement to other medical technologies, and thus the higher cost (or diminished effectiveness) of antibiotics lowers the value of other medical technologies. No one has yet estimated this indirect cost, but it could well dwarf the direct costs of antibiotic resistance.

Many studies have documented longer hospital stays and increased costs for medication and care associated with resistant pathogens. The situation where an infection does not respond to any known antibiotic is becoming increasingly common. Since death is the likely outcome, the costs of contracting such a multidrug-resistant strain are likely to be much greater than current estimates.

Quantifying the health and economic impacts of resistance has proven to be a significant though surmountable research challenge. In hospital settings, the challenge has been disentangling two effects: the longer the hospital stay, the greater the likelihood of being infected with a resistant pathogen, and in turn, a hospital-acquired infection with a resistant pathogen lengthens the hospital stay. In community settings, the challenge has been correctly estimating both the benefits and the costs of antibiotic use. Resistance-related costs alone are insufficient reason to recommend that fewer antibiotics be used, since antibiotics bring benefits as well as costs. To date, there has been no reliable benefit-cost estimate of antibiotic use in either setting.

The scale of the resistance problem may be self-evident to those in the medical and public health communities who deal with it on a daily basis. However, assessing the economic impact at a national scale is a necessary first step to bring the problem to the attention of policymakers and stakeholders, including purchasers of health insurance and government agencies like the Center for Medicare and Medicaid Services.

# References

**Abboud, F. M. and B. A. Waisbren. (1959).** "Correlation Between in Vitro Studies and Response to Antibiotic Therapy in Staphylococcic Bacteremia." *Archives of Internal Medicine* 104(2): 226-33.

**Arakawa, Y., Y. Ike, et al. (2000).** "Trends in Antimicrobial-Drug Resistance in Japan." *Emerging Infectious Diseases* 6(6).

**Archer, G. L. (1998).** "*Staphylococcus aureus:* A Well-Armed Pathogen." *Clinical Infectious Diseases* 26(5): 1179-81.

**Arias, C. A., J. Reyes, et al. (2003).** "Multicentre Surveillance of Antimicrobial Resistance in Enterococci and Staphylococci from Colombian Hospitals, 2001-2002." *The Journal of Antimicrobial Chemotherapy* 51(1): 59-68.

**Armstrong, G. L., L. A. Conn, et al. (1999).** "Trends in Infectious Disease Mortality in the United States During the 20th Century." *JAMA* 281(1): 61-6.

**Bantar, C., A. Famiglietti, et al. (2004).** "Análisis de los Dos Cortes de Prevalencia de los Años 2002 y 2003 [Comparative Analysis During Two Periods of Prevalence from 1999 to 2003]." Bulletins 144, 153, 158, and 167. (In Spanish) Asociación Argentina de Microbiología, Buenos Aires, Argentina. http://www.aam.org.ar/archivos/167_SIR .pdf (accessed May 31, 2006).

**Blot, S.I., K.H. Vandewoude, et al. (2002).** "Outcome and Attributable Mortality in Critically Ill Patients with Bacteremia Involving Methicillin-Susceptible and Methicillin-Resistant *Staphylococcus aureus.*" *Archives of Internal Medicine* 162: 2229-2235.

**Bouchillon, S. K., B. M. Johnson, et al. (2004).** "Determining Incidence of Extended Spectrum [Beta]-Lactamase Producing *Enterobacteriaceae,* Vancomycin-Resistant *Enterococcus faecium* and Methicillin-Resistant *Staphylococcus aureus* in 38 Centres from 17 Countries: the PEARLS Study 2001-2002." *International Journal of Antimicrobial Agents* 24(2): 119-124.

**Briggs, S., A. Upton, et al. (2002).** "Vancomycin-Resistant Enterococcal Colonisation of Hospitalised Patients in Auckland [Abstract Only]." *The New Zealand Medical Journal.* 115(1160): U145.

**CDC (1993).** "Nosocomial Enterococci Resistant to Vancomycin— United States, 1989-1993." *MMWR. Morbidity and Mortality Weekly Report* 42(30): 597-9. Centers for Disease Control and Prevention.

**——. (1999).** "National Nosocomial Infections Surveillance (NNIS) System Report, Data Summary from January 1990-May 1999, Issued June 1999." *American Journal of Infection Control* 27(6): 520-532.

**——. (2000).** "National Nosocomial Infections Surveillance (NNIS) System Report, Data Summary from January 1992-April 2000, Issued June 2000." *American Journal of Infection Control* 28(6): 429-448.

**——. (2001).** "National Nosocomial Infections Surveillance (NNIS) System Report, Data Summary from January 1992-June 2001, Issued August 2001." *American Journal of Infection Control* 29(6): 404-421.

**——. (2003).** "National Nosocomial Infections Surveillance (NNIS) System Report, Data Summary from January 1992 Through June 2003, Issued August 2003." *American Journal of Infection Control* 31(8): 481-498.

**——. (2004).** "National Nosocomial Infections Surveillance (NNIS) System Report, Data Summary from January 1992 Through June 2004, Issued October 2004." *American Journal of Infection Control* 32(8): 470-485.

**Chang, S. and D.M. Sievert. (2003).** "Infection with Vancomycin-Resistant *Staphylococcus aureus* Containing the vanA Resistance Gene." *The New England Journal of Medicine* 348(14): 1342-1347.

**Cizman, M., B. Beovic, et al. (2004).** "Antibiotic Policies in Central Eastern Europe." *International Journal of Antimicrobial Agents* 24(3): 199-204.

**Cosgrove, S.E., Y. Qi, et al. (2005).** "The Impact of Methicillin Resistance in *Staphylococcus aureus* Bacteremia on Patient Outcomes: Mortality, Length of Stay, and Hospital Charges." *Infection Control and Hospital Epidemiology* 26: 166-174.

**Diekema, D. J., M. A. Pfaller, et al. (2000).** "Trends in Antimicrobial Susceptibility of Bacterial Pathogens Isolated from Patients with Bloodstream Infections in the USA, Canada and Latin America." *International Journal of Antimicrobial Agents* 13(4): 257-271.

**Elbasha, E. H. (2003).** "Deadweight Loss of Bacterial Resistance Due to Overtreatment." *Health Economics* 12(2): 125-38.

**GAO (1999).** *Antimicrobial Resistance: Data to Assess Public Health Threat From Resistant Bacteria Are Limited.* GAO/HEHS/NSIAD/ RCED-99-132. http://www.gao.gov/archive/1999/hx99132.pdf (accessed May 31, 2006). U.S. General Accounting Office.

Gaynes, R. and J. R. Edwards. (2005). "Overview of Nosocomial Infections Caused by Gram-Negative Bacilli." *Clinical Infectious Diseases* 41(6): 848-54.

Goossens, H., M. Ferech, et al. (2003). "European Surveillance of Antibiotic Consumption (ESAC) Interactive Database." http://www.esac.ua.ac.be (accessed January 20, 2006).

Herold, B. C., L. C. Immergluck, et al. (1998). "Community-Acquired Methicillin-Resistant *Staphylococcus aureus* in Children with No Identified Predisposing Risk." *JAMA* 279(8): 593-8.

Ho, P. L. F. (2003). "Carriage of Methicillin-Resistant *Staphylococcus aureus*, Ceftazidime-Resistant Gram-Negative Bacilli, and Vancomycin-Resistant Enterococci Before and After Intensive Care Unit Admission." *Critical Care Medicine* 31(4): 1175-1182.

Holmberg, S. D., S. L. Solomon, et al. (1987). "Health and Economic Impacts of Antimicrobial Resistance." *Reviews of Infectious Diseases* 9(Nov.-Dec.): 1065-78.

Howard, D. and K. Rask. (2002). The Impact of Resistance on Antibiotic Demand in Patients with Ear Infections. *Battling Resistance to Antibiotics and Pesticides: An Economic Approach*. R. Laxminarayan (ed.). Washington, DC: RFF Press, 119-133.

Jones, M., D. Draghi, et al. (2004). "Emerging Resistance Among Bacterial Pathogens in the Intensive Care Unit: A European and North American Surveillance Study (2000-2002)." *Annals of Clinical Microbiology and Antimicrobials* 3(14).

Kim, T., P.I. Oh, et al. (2001). "The Economic Impact of Methicillin-Resistant *Staphylococcus aureus* in Canadian Hospitals." *Infection Control and Hospital Epidemiology* 22(2): 99-104.

Klein, E., R. Laxminarayan. (2006). "Hospitalizations and Deaths in the U.S. Due to Vancomycin-Resistant Enterococcal and Methicillin-resistant *Staphylococcus aureus* Infections, 2004." Working paper. Washington, DC: Resources for the Future.

Klein, E., D. L. Smith, et al. (2007). "Trends in Hospitalizations and Deaths in the U.S. due to *Staphylococcus aureus* and MRSA Infections, 1999-2004." Manuscript submitted for publication.

Kuehnert, M. J., H. A. Hill, et al. (2005). "Methicillin-Resistant *Staphylococcus aureus* Hospitalizations, United States." *Emerging Infectious Diseases* 11(6): 868-72.

Lee, K., Y. A. Kim, et al. (2004). "Increasing Prevalence of Vancomycin-Resistant Enterococci, and Cefoxitin-, Imipenem- and Fluoroquinolone-Resistant Gram-Negative Bacilli: A KONSAR Study in 2002." *Yonsei Medical Journal* 45(4): 598-608.

Liu, G., S. Xu, et al. (2003). "Analysis of Antimicrobial Resistance of Clinical Isolates of Enterococci from Beijing and Other Areas in China [Article in Chinese Abstract Only]." *Zhonghua Yi Xue Za Zhi* 83(12): 1049-52.

Lowy, F. D. (1998). "*Staphylococcus aureus* Infections." *The New England Journal of Medicine* 339(8): 520-532.

Matsumoto, T., T. Muratani, et al. (2004). "No Regional Spread of Vancomycin-Resistant Enterococci with vanA or vanB in Kitakyushu, Japan." *Journal of Infection and Chemotherapy* 10(6): 331-334.

McDonald, L. C. (2006). "Trends in Antimicrobial Resistance in Health Care-Associated Pathogens and Effect on Treatment." *Clinical Infectious Diseases* 42(S2): S65-S71.

McDonald, L. C., T. L. Lauderdale, et al. (2004). "The Status of Antimicrobial Resistance in Taiwan Among Gram-Positive Pathogens: the Taiwan Surveillance of Antimicrobial Resistance (TSAR) Programme, 2000." *International Journal of Antimicrobial Agents* 23(4): 362-370.

McManus, P., M. L. Hammond, et al. (1997). "Antibiotic Use in the Australian Community, 1990-1995." *The Medical Journal of Australia* 167(3): 124-7.

Melo, M. C. N., M. C. Silva-Carvalho, et al. (2004). "Detection and Molecular Characterization of a Gentamicin-Susceptible, Methicillin-Resistant *Staphylococcus aureus* (MRSA) Clone in Rio de Janeiro that Resembles the New York/Japanese Clone." *Journal of Hospital Infection* 58(4): 276-285.

National Prescribing Service. (2005). "Antibiotic Prescribing Is Increasingly Judicious." *National Prescribing Service Newsletter* 40(June). http://www.nps.org.au/resources/NPS_News/news40/news40.pdf (accessed May 31, 2006).

Nimmo, G. R., J. M. Bell, et al. (2003). "Fifteen Years of Surveillance by the Australian Group for Antimicrobial Resistance (AGAR)." *Communicable Diseases Intelligence* 27 Suppl: S47-54.

Noskin, G.A., R.J. Rubin, et al. (2005). "The Burden of *Staphylococcus aureus* Infections on Hospitals in the United States: An Analysis of the 2000 and 2001 Nationwide Inpatient Sample Database." *Archives of Internal Medicine* 165(15): 1756-1761.

Osmon, S., D. Warren, et al. (2003). "The Influence of Infection on Hospital Mortality for Patients Requiring > 48 h of Intensive Care." *Chest* 124(3): 1021-9.

OTA. (1995). *Impact of Antibiotic-Resistant Bacteria: A Report to the U.S. Congress.* Washington, DC: Government Printing Office. Office of Technology Assessment.

Palumbi, S.R. (2001). "Humans as the World's Greatest Evolutionary Force." *Science* 293(5536): 1786-1790.

Phelps, C. E. (1989). "Bug/Drug Resistance: Sometimes Less Is More." *Medical Care* 27(2): 194-203.

RIVM. (2005). "European Antimicrobial Resistance Surveillance System (EARSS)." http://www.rivm.nl/earss (accessed January 18, 2005). The National Institute for Public Health and the Environment.

Rubin, R. J., C. A. Harrington, et al. (1999). "The Economic Impact of *Staphylococcus aureus* in New York City Hospitals." *Emerging Infectious Diseases* 5(1): 9-17.

Skinner, D. and C. S. Keefer. (1941). "Significance of Bacteremia Caused by *Staphylococcus aureus.*" *Archives of Internal Medicine* 68: 851-75.

Steinman, M. A., R. Gonzales, et al. (2003). "Changing Use of Antibiotics in Community-Based Outpatient Practice, 1991–1999." *Annals of Internal Medicine* 138: 525-533.

The Genesis Report. (1994). The Real War on Drugs: Bacteria Are Winning. New Jersey.

Titze-de-Almeida, R., M. R. Filho, et al. (2004). "Molecular Epidemiology and Antimicrobial Susceptibility of Enterococci Recovered from Brazilian Intensive Care Units." *The Brazilian Journal of Infectious Diseases* 8(3): 197-205.

Udo, E. E., N. Al-Sweih, et al. (2003). "Species Prevalence and Antibacterial Resistance of Enterococci Isolated in Kuwait Hospitals." *Journal of Medical Microbiology* 52(2): 163-168.

Weinstein, R. A. (2003). "Antibiotic Resistance in Hospitals and Intensive Care Units: the Problem and Potential Solutions." *Seminars in Respiratory and Critical Care Medicine* 24(1): 113-20.

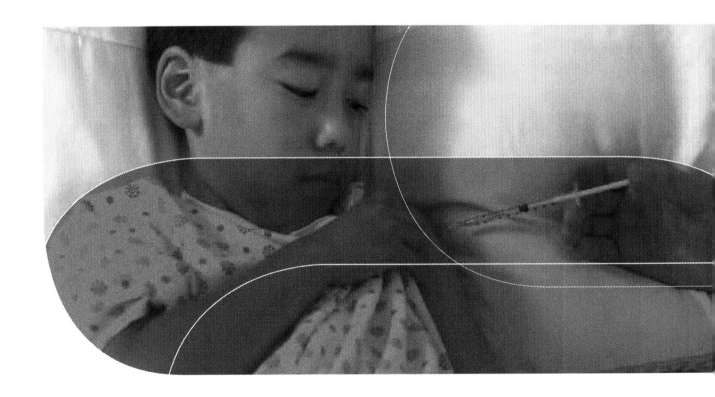

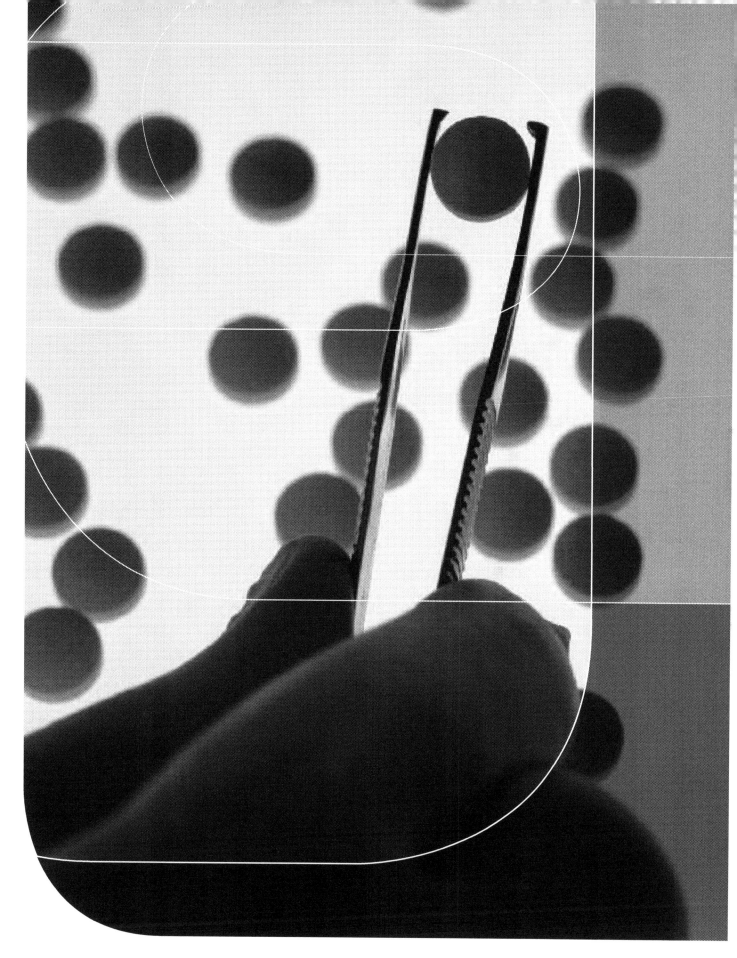

# CHAPTER 2

# The epidemiology of antibiotic resistance: **Policy levers**

*David L. Smith*

The evolution of antibiotic resistance is defined as a change in the frequency of bacterial genes that affects the way bacteria populations respond to antibiotics, including their ability to grow at different drug concentrations and to persist through antibiotic chemotherapy. Ultimately, these genetic changes lower the effectiveness of antibiotic medicines and increase the length and cost of hospital stays, the probability of treatment failure, and the incidence of severe complications, such as chronic sequelae or death (Carbon 1999; Rubin, Harrington et al. 1999). This chapter focuses on the biological and epidemiological context for the evolution of antibiotic resistance and the policy levers that can be pulled to slow or possibly reverse the spread of resistance.

The biological study of antibiotic resistance spans many academic disciplines that are concerned with phenomena at, below, or above the level of a single bacterial cell. Cellular and molecular phenomena are relevant for finding new compounds to develop into drugs and for understanding the cellular and genetic mechanisms of resistance and cross resistance—that is, resistance to several drugs that is conferred by a single genetic mechanism (Box 2.1). These phenomena set the stage for understanding the evolution of resistance, but cellular and molecular phenomena are only distantly related to risk and cannot be manipulated through policy; it is hard to imagine a policy that would target individual cells, except for chemotherapy itself.

Our focus is on those aspects of the biology that are directly related to changes in risk and can be affected through policy—typically phenomena above the level of a cell, such as population dynamics and control. The evolution of resistance

**BOX 2.1**

## DEFINING FUNCTIONAL RESISTANCE GROUPS

The current definition of what constitutes a new or different "class" of antibiotics (macrolides, cephalosporins, etc.) is based on the chemical structure of the active molecule of an antibiotic. The problem is that there is often an inconsistency between this method of classifying antibiotics and the goal of promoting the effectiveness of antibiotics. Use of an antibiotic in one chemical class could select for a resistance mechanism that also confers resistance to an antibiotic in a different chemical class while having little bearing on resistance to other antibiotics within the same chemical class. Because resistance is the biggest threat to antibiotic effectiveness, it is a more useful characteristic around which to organize antibiotics.

To facilitate thinking about different groups of antibiotics as distinct resource pools, we propose grouping antibiotics into functional resistance groups (FRGs). The logic is the same as that applied to natural resources. Oil, for example, is grouped into "deposits" based on physical contiguity because only when two companies drill the same deposit will they have a negative externality on one another. Two or more antibiotics can be defined as belonging to the same FRG if the use of one antibiotic in that FRG generates resistance to the other antibiotics in the same FRG, but not to antibiotics in other FRGs.

The mechanisms that define FRGs are those that play a role in the emergence and spread of antibiotic resistance: the mode of action by the antibiotic and the mechanism by which the bacteria evades the antibiotic. The mechanism of action employed by the antibiotic is one aspect. For example, one group of antibiotics (including penicillin and cephalosporins) may interfere with biosynthesis of cell walls in Gram-positive bacteria, another group (including quinolones and 2-pyridones) may prevent DNA replication in bacteria by interfering with the uncoiling of chromosomes, and yet a third group (including tetracylines) may thwart DNA replication by simply inhibiting protein biosynthesis. The nature of a bacterial strain's response to these antibiotics is the mechanism that defines FRGs. For example, *E. coli* has developed a gene that codes for a protein called TetA that literally pumps tetracycline molecules out of the bacterium. This "efflux pump" also removes other molecules, so it confers resistance to chemically unrelated antibiotics. FRGs are not likely to overlap with chemical classes, since resistance to different antibiotics conferred by different genes can be contained on a single mobile genetic element, such as a plasmid or chromosomal cassette.

There may be practical problems in defining FRGs, but similar problems in resistance have been surmounted with careful expert assessment, such as the problem of deciding how to translate laboratory tests for resistance into useful clinical criteria. A more serious challenge is that the definition of an FRG may not be static. Cross-resistance may spread across antibiotics, and its scope may vary across countries. Moreover, the extent of cross-resistance may differ across bacterial species. Therefore, FRGs may change over time and space and may need to be species-specific. Despite these difficulties, many of the basic concepts that would define FRGs already exist in practice. The immediate task is to sharpen the definition of FRGs and use them in a more formal way.

Many "new" antibiotics belong to the same chemical classes as old antibiotics. To be patented, they must differ significantly from existing antibiotics, but "different" is defined by the rules of intellectual property. For example, new drugs might have a better safety profile than old ones. New drugs are often identical to existing drugs, however, from the perspective of resistance. The evolution of antibiotic resistance to two or more antibiotic drugs whose patents are held by different companies undermines any economic incentives that a company might have to manage antibiotics to minimize the spread of resistance. Resistance becomes a common property problem for the companies (see Chapter 7).

To regulate antibiotics for antibiotic resistance, it may be necessary to identify groups of antibiotics that are functionally related. Ideally, two antibiotics would belong to the same group if the same gene conferred resistance to both drugs. In reality, it is difficult to define functional groups. A single gene can change a bacterial clone's resistance profile to several antibiotics all at once. Some resistance mechanisms, such as an efflux pump, are so broad that they confer high-level resistance to chemically unrelated antibiotics, and resistance to multiple antibiotics conferred by different genes can be contained on a single mobile genetic element, such as a plasmid or chromosomal cassette. Functional groups, moreover, might be defined differently for different bacteria species.

Despite the practical difficulties of formally defining functional resistance groups, the concept already exists in practice. The mechanisms that define FRGs clearly play some role in the emergence and spread of antibiotic resistance, and therefore are as important for studying resistance as they are for regulating it.

—Laxminarayan, Malani, & Smith

and the associated increased risks of treatment failure involve not just the mechanisms that confer resistance to antibiotics, but also the likelihood that some bacteria are resistant to chemotherapy, regardless of the biological mechanism. The cell-level conceptual divide does not always cleanly delimit the relevant subjects; for example, the movement of plasmids among bacteria is a subcellular phenomenon with population-level consequences. The important distinction is whether the biological process is related to changing risk within some population of interest.

The approach here is eclectic; we borrow from many academic disciplines that are concerned with population-level phenomena, including ecology, microbial ecology, population biology, infectious disease epidemiology, evolutionary biology, and population genetics. Changes in risk are quantitative phenomena, so the study of antibiotic resistance inevitably involves some sort of mathematical model. Mathematical models of the spread of antibiotic resistance help synthesize information from multiple disciplines, and they are important conceptual tools for evaluating control measures (Box 2.2). This chapter begins by describing the biological background for the problem and then proceeds to the policy levers that can be pulled to change the biological world.

The concepts that are important for understanding the evolution of antibiotic resistance and its control are the ecology and structure of bacteria populations, the epidemiology of infection, the treatment of an infection, and the origins and spread of resistant bacteria. This chapter discusses each of these concepts in turn. We then examine the goals of controlling resistance and define an appropriate aim—to maximize the total net benefit of antibiotics in a population over time. Once the goal is articulated, we can look at strategies for achieving it: controlling antibiotic use, controlling infections, and pursuing interesting new approaches based in ecology. Finally, we review some success stories and identify common threads.

**BOX 2.2**

## MATHEMATICAL MODELS FOR STUDYING RESISTANCE

The evolution of resistance is often studied using mathematical models. Mathematical models are necessary in the study of infectious diseases because the infection process is not directly observable, because humans are not readily subject to experimentation for practical and ethical reasons, and because the assumptions of ordinary statistical tests are often violated for infectious diseases (Becker 1989). Several types of mathematical models are relevant.

*PK/PD models.* Pharmacokinetic (PK) and pharmacodynamic (PD) models are primarily used to help design the frequency, dose, and duration of chemotherapy to ensure that the drugs cure an infection while simultaneously limiting toxic side effects at high drug concentrations. PK models focus on drug kinetics—changes in the concentration of the drug over time in the active sites, including infected tissues and affected tissues where toxicity is a concern. PD models focus on the population dynamics of the pathogen in response to the drug kinetics—the net effect of the drug on the pathogen population. PK/PD models help ensure that the concentrations of antibiotic at the active site are high enough for long enough to eliminate an infection, especially between doses, when drug concentrations the drop. Evolution of the bacteria population during antibiotic chemotherapy is an increasingly important cause of treatment failure. To improve chemotherapy and manage resistance, some PK/PD models are now considering the evolution of resistance (Drusano 2003; Drusano 2005).

*Models for the evolution of de novo resistance.* The evolution of resistance during treatment takes on a new significance if the pathogen can spread to other hosts. The evolution of a resistant pathogen with the capability of spreading may involve several genetic changes; meanwhile, the newly evolved drug-resistant pathogen persists and continues to evolve despite intense competition with drug-sensitive pathogens. Such antibiotic-resistant bacteria are one kind of emerging pathogen, and the paradigm for other emerging pathogens, such as Ebola or the 1918 flu. Using mathematical models provides some important insights into *de novo* emergence (Antia, Regoes et al. 2003). The emerging pathogen paradigm provides a useful conceptual link between PK/PD models and epidemiological models.

*Epidemiological models.* Epidemiological models are concerned with the spread of resistance within a population of hosts, especially the transmission of a resistant pathogen from one host to another (Austin, Kakehashi et al. 1997; Austin, Kristinsson et al. 1999; Cooper, Medley et al. 1999; Smith, Dushoff et al. 2004). Epidemiological models are useful conceptually, to help understand the factors that affect the spread of resistance, and for evaluating control measures (Bonhoeffer, Lipsitch et al. 1997; Bergstrom, Lo et al. 2004; Cooper, Medley et al. 2004). Because the assumptions of standard statistical models are violated for infectious diseases, including antibiotic-resistant pathogens, mathematical models are increasingly being used to design, analyze, and interpret studies (Lipsitch, Bergstrom et al. 2000; Pelupessy, Bonten et al. 2002).

## Structure of bacteria populations

To describe changes in the frequency of resistance within a population, it is first necessary to define a population, but this is not an easy task. Bacteria populations and communities have a complex distribution and functional structure. One natural definition of a bacteria population is all the bacteria of a single species within a single host or part of a host. Another is all the bacteria that are shared among a well-defined population of hosts. Both definitions are relevant for the epidemiology of resistance. Within any single human, bacteria populations come and go, but even as the local population is subject to turnover, the bacteria population in a collection of hosts is stable because of transmission or colonization from other hosts. In ecology, structured populations that are characterized by local demographic instability but global stability through recolonization are called metapopulations.

The emergence of resistant bacteria within a single host and the spread of resistant bacteria or genes (McGowan 1983; Davies 1994) among hosts are closely interrelated processes, and substantial research has been directed at understanding the interplay between the processes that occur within and among hosts (Levin 2001; Lipsitch 2001). Most host populations, moreover, have their own spatial distribution and contact network, and this imposes a higher-order structure on bacteria populations (Smith, Dushoff et al. 2004). Bacteria can also have an important reservoir outside, in a nonhuman host or the environment (Kummerer 2004). Since bacteria spread within and among hosts and even shift host species, the proper definition of a bacteria population is determined by the question at hand and by the temporal and spatial scale that it implies.

For bacteria, humans are one kind of habitat. The bacteria populations within a single human host have a particular niche, a mode of life in some part of the body where they are typically found in healthy people. For many bacteria species, the gut is the primary habitat. Other important microbial communities in humans are found in the mouth and nose, the skin, the ear, and the vaginal tract. Most of the time, the bacteria populations in these habitats are harmless to their host, and some are beneficial. Bacteria populations that persist on a host asymptomatically are said to colonize a host, and the host is said to be a carrier. Colonization with commensal bacteria, even resistant bacteria, is not generally regarded as an important medical phenomenon per se. Colonization with bacteria is a natural, necessary, and inevitable condition of life.

> Colonization with bacteria is a natural, necessary, and inevitable condition of life.

Bacteria, including resistant bacteria, become a medical problem when they cause an infection—the invasion of tissues where bacteria are not normally found, such as the bloodstream, lungs, urinary tract, other sterile sites of the body, or wounds. For example, enterococci are commonly found in the gut, but they can cause a life-threatening infection when they enter the bloodstream, often through a wound, and begin to proliferate. Infection is generally accompanied by some symptoms, but the line between colonization and infection is sometimes fuzzy.

Colonizing bacteria compete with other bacteria of the same species and of different species for the habitat they occupy. The bacteria communities that inhabit an individual human are some mix of stable flora, bacteria that persist in the host

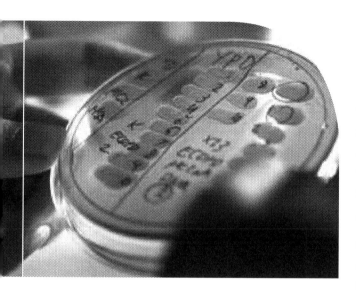

the interactions with other bacteria, bacteria may be subject to infections themselves. Some viruses, called bacteriophages, invade bacteria populations sporadically and limit or eliminate their populations. Infections by other parasites can change the community indirectly, mediated through an immune response that changes the flora or through antimicrobial use. Most of these processes are poorly studied but contribute to the enormous variability in bacterial flora over time, including sporadic changes to the "stable" flora.

The perturbations caused by antibiotic use are the most important factor in the evolution of antibiotic resistance. Antibiotics eliminate sensitive bacteria and open up niches for resistant bacteria or other species to grow, and they can also cause wholesale changes to the gut, such as antibiotic-associated diarrhea. Another effect is bacterial overgrowth—a rapid increase in the bacterial load of some species, a side effect of eliminating other species with antibiotics (Donskey, Hanrahan et al. 1999; Donskey, Chowdhry et al. 2000; Donskey, Hanrahan et al. 2000). During these periods of perturbation, the bacterial clones that make up the transient flora may expand and find a more permanent place within the gut. Such events may be important for helping antibiotic-resistant bacteria become a part of the stable flora, thereby making the host a carrier.

An important but often overlooked principle is that antibiotic use selects for resistance in several different species of bacteria simultaneously, regardless of the reasons why a patient takes the drug. When a patient takes an antibiotic to treat an infection, the concentrations of that antibiotic become elevated and affect target as well as non-target species, including bacteria from many microhabitats throughout the body. The mode of administering the antibiotic does have some effect because it affects the concentrations of the drug in other parts of the body; antibiotics typically reach much higher concentrations in the gut if given orally rather than intravenously (Drusano 2005).

for years, and transient flora—bacteria that were recently acquired and that are just passing through. The stability of bacterial flora may be due to persistence in refugia inside the body—surfaces to which they may adhere or that otherwise protect them from other microbes or the immune system.

Many factors affect the composition of the stable bacterial flora that inhabit a host. Bacteria colonize the body within the first few days of life. Most bacteria produce some metabolic by-products that alter the environment; these chemicals may help construct a niche in their local environment that favors them, a niche that could last throughout the life of the host. The immune system and physical environment combine to shape the bacterial flora. Immune chemicals act as a sort of top-down regulation that influences the composition of the microbial community. Similar principles apply to the fine-grain-structure body surfaces where bacteria adhere.

Bacteria compete with one another indirectly by consuming scarce resources, and directly through a sort of chemical warfare, or by changing the chemical composition of the surrounding environment (Dykes 1995; Jack, Tagg et al. 1995; Dykes and Hastings 1997; Riley and Wertz 2002). On top of

All this suggests that the human body is a highly dynamic and variable environment. Given this unpredictability, no host is likely to provide a stable home forever. Thus, bacteria's mode of life within a host is only one component of bacterial fitness. To persist within a population of hosts over time, bacteria must spread to other hosts. The spread of bacteria (and resistant bacteria) that stabilizes bacteria metapopulations is a largely invisible process involving colonization of healthy humans, with occasional infection. A human population represents a bacteria metapopulation with a particular kind of structure (i.e., the spatial distribution and contact network of the hosts) that affects the way bacteria spread.

Epidemiologically important contact occurs as a part of normal life. Opportunities for spread are more common among people who are frequently in contact, including family members, coworkers, schoolmates, or members of a church or health club. Other important types of structure include hospitals, where health care workers act as vectors, and more structure is added by the exchange of patients among hospitals, long-term care facilities, and the surrounding community (Trick, Kuehnert et al. 1999; Smith, Dushoff et al. 2004). Also associated with the spread of antibiotic-resistant bacteria are intravenous drug use (Saravolatz, Markowitz et al. 1982; Saravolatz, Pohlod et al. 1982) and prison populations (Aiello, Lowy et al. 2006). Typically, bacteria spread to those people with whom contact occurs most often, but eventually, bacteria can spread among less connected populations. At regional, national, and global levels, resistant bacteria spread through international business and travel (Okeke and Edelman 2001; O'Brien 2002). The structures of human population that determine contact work together with the natural changes in bacterial flora within a body, thus providing opportunity for bacteria (including resistant bacteria) to spread among populations.

The complement of transmission is persistence: the among-host component of bacterial fitness is the product of the rate at which bacteria are transmitted to other hosts per day and the number of days that the bacteria persist. In other words, bacteria can increase their among-host component of fitness by spreading more efficiently, or by persisting in a host and "shedding"[1] for a longer period of time. One of the important fitness effects of antibiotics is to shorten the persistence times of sensitive bacteria by depressing their among-host fitness relative to antibiotic-resistant bacteria. In some cases, colonization with antibiotic-resistant bacteria is extremely persistent; a carrier can shed the same bacteria for years (Bonten, Hayden et al. 1996; Henning, Delencastre et al. 1996). In fact carriers have been shown to play a special role in epidemics (Smith, Dushoff et al. 2004). The efficiency of control might be vastly improved by finding and targeting carriers—by isolation during hospitalization or selective decontamination (see discussion below).

From a medical-ecological perspective, bacteria differ in many ways: their niche, their propensity to colonize and infect humans, their effect on human health, their ability to spread among humans, and the severity of symptoms when they cause disease. The antibiotic resistance problem in the United States is split between hospital-acquired and community-acquired pathogens; most of the bacteria are hospital acquired except for *Streptococcus pneumonia* (a.k.a. pneumococci) and a recently emerged community-acquired *Staphylococcus aureus*. Antibiotic resistance is common in both Gram-negative bacteria and Gram-positive bacteria, such as staphylococci, streptococci, and enterococci.

■

## Epidemiology of infection

When bacteria infect an ordinarily sterile site, they present a serious medical condition, even if they are not resistant to

---

1   For bacteria to reach other hosts, they must be shed from carriers. Shedding means that bacteria are broadcast into the environment surrounding a host.

antibiotics. To understand bacterial infections, it is important to characterize the source: where were the progenitors of the infecting bacteria a few generations previously? Here, we give an epidemiological, ecological, non-clinical overview of bacterial infections and the ecological reservoir.

Perhaps the most important ecological reservoir for an infection is the population of bacteria that colonize some other part of the host's body. The most common route of infection is the spread of bacteria from one part of a host's body to another, moved around by the host itself or by a caregiver. In many cases, the infection starts from contamination with colonizing flora during a medical procedure.

In other cases, the bacterial infection is spread from other hosts, including other hospital patients, hospital workers, family members, or schoolmates (Bonten, Slaughter et al. 1998). The relative importance of these host reservoirs as a source of infection probably declines as a function of proximity to the focal host; the most likely sources are the patients themselves, followed by health care workers, other hospital patients, and family members.

The bacteria are transmitted by direct contact, such as touching or sneezing, or indirect contact through an intermediate contaminated object (a "fomite"). For example, health care workers can be carriers, or they may be vectors who move bacteria among patients or from contaminated objects in a patient's room. The objects that surround individuals, including furniture and food and water, can become contaminated. Medical devices are a particularly important source of infections (Lund, Agvald-Ohman et al. 2002; Agvald-Ohman, Lund et al. 2004): they bring a potentially contaminated surface into contact with living tissue. One problem with medical devices is that their wet surfaces facilitate the growth of biofilms (Box 2.3), which can help facilitate gene exchange and persistence, protect bacteria from antibiotics, and so provide a natural refuge and gentle exposure that may become important in the evolution of resistance (Costerton, Stewart et al. 1999).

A potential source of antibiotic resistance in environmental bacteria is the sewage effluent from hospitals and long-term care facilities, which contains large numbers of resistant bacteria (Kummerer 2004). Large amounts of antibiotics are also used in agriculture for prophylaxis or as nutritional supplements, and antibiotic-resistant bacteria can remain in meat through the abattoir and retail (Witte 1998). Most meat is properly cooked in the home or in restaurants, but uncooked meat can cross-contaminate raw foods during preparation. This is a potentially important source of exposure and perhaps colonization. Like hospital sewage, the effluent from farms that use antibiotics can be a source

## BOX 2.3

### BIOFILMS ON MEDICAL DEVICES

A biofilm is a community of surface-adherent bacteria embedded in an extracellular matrix composed of protein, polysaccharides, and nucleic acids (Costerton, Stewart et al. 1999; Fux, Stoodley et al. 2003). Biofilms are often found on wet surfaces, including teeth and water tubing. Biofilms on medical devices are extremely persistent and naturally resistant to antibiotics and thus contribute to the incidence of device-associated bacterial infections. Resistance in biofilms is different from evolved resistance, but it may play a role in the evolution of resistance by facilitating gene exchange and by providing an environment where bacteria are exposed to gentle doses of antibiotics. Bacteria with evolved resistance can also be found in biofilms, especially in hospitals.

## AGRICULTURAL ANTIBIOTIC USE, ZOONOTIC PATHOGENS, AND ZOONOTIC ORIGINS OF RESISTANCE

Common causes of diarrhea are *Campylobacter jejuni* and *Salmonella* species. These are called zoonotic pathogens because they are usually acquired from animals and not generally transmitted among humans. Antibiotic resistance in zoonotic infections is generally attributed to the use of antibiotics in agriculture, especially fluoroquinolones, although the fraction attributable to agricultural antibiotic use has been controversial (e.g., see Phillips, Casewell et al. 2004 and the associated correspondence).

Part of the rise in the frequency of antibiotic resistance in hospital- and community-acquired pathogens may be attributable to the use of antibiotics in agriculture, so reductions in the amount of antibiotics used on farms may reduce the emergence of new types of antibiotic resistance. Agricultural use of antibiotics may contribute to clinically important antibiotic resistance in ways that are both important and hard to demonstrate (Smith, Dushoff et al. 2005). For example, farms may be the source of new resistance genes that move across species and into humans to initiate epidemics (Courvalin 2000; Smith, Harris et al. 2002). Alternatively, farms can be a continuous source of resistance genes, but this would be less important than medical antibiotic use if the latter was the primary driver for resistance. For zoonotic bacteria, however, human-to-human transmission is rare, and for these species, antibiotic resistance in infections in humans must be related to the reservoir of resistance in the zoonotic reservoir, or to some unidentified and nonpathogenic reservoir of resistance genes in the humans. In any case, the European Union has banned the use of antibiotics for growth promotion, and the U.S. Food and Drug Administration recently withdrew its approval of fluoroquinolones based on the human health concern of antibiotic resistance, and approval of new antibiotics for agricultural use will require an assessment of the risks to human health.

of antibiotic-resistant bacteria in the environment (Witte 1998). Alternatively, farmers may become colonized by novel strains of antibiotic-resistant bacteria and transmit them into the population (Aubry-Damon, Grenet et al. 2004). Other sources of bacterial infections are the animals themselves. Infections with zoonotic pathogens are typically acquired from contact with animal food products or animals, usually without subsequent transmission to other humans (Box 2.4).

The human body is constantly bombarded by bacteria, but most potential bacterial infections are prevented by the immune system (Levin and Antia 2001). Infections often begin when the immune system is compromised. The skin provides the first and most important protection, but wounds compromise immune protection and allow bacteria to gain access to blood and other tissues. The risk of infection is further exacerbated when medical devices contaminated with biofilms bring the bacterial world into close contact with ordinarily sterile sites, especially the insertion of intravenous needles and tubes to aid with breathing or urination.

In patients with compromised immune systems, including the elderly, patients with HIV/AIDS, cancer or transplant patients, and patients who have recently had influenza, bacterial infections have become increasingly common. Such patients constitute an important segment of the population at risk from antibiotic-resistant infections. Their compromised immune status and multiple health problems make computing the burden of disease for antibiotic resistance difficult.

Bacterial infections grow exponentially at first, so a small initial population of bacteria cells can threaten a patient's life within a few days. The longer a bacterial infection continues without treatment, the higher the peak bacteria population densities, the greater the genetic diversity, and the greater the risk of complications (Paterson and Rice 2003). Left untreated, acute bacterial infections can develop into chronic infections when bacteria adhere to body tissues (Fux, Stoodley et al. 2003).

■
―――――――――――――――――――――――――――

## Treatment of infection

Not all infections need antibiotics, not all are curable by antibiotics, and not all treatment failures are due to evolved resistance. Once an infection begins, the immune system mounts a response that limits or clears an infection. Antibiotic treatment, however, substantially limits the duration and severity of the infection, especially when the immune response is insufficient. Antibiotic therapy often shortens the duration of symptoms and decreases the likelihood of complications and death.

All else equal, the earlier an effective antibiotic is given during the course of an infection, the better the prognosis for a successful recovery. Since infections grow exponentially, at least initially, the earlier antibiotics are used, the less work they have to do. When a patient presents with symptoms that resemble a bacterial infection, a doctor who suspects a bacterial infection on the basis of her initial diagnosis usually chooses an antibiotic without a microbiological confirmation of the infecting agent. This method for selecting antibiotics, called empiric therapy, is common practice. Since antibiotics are most effective if they are used immediately, empiric therapy is preferred, and it is probably good for patients (Paterson and Rice 2003). On the other hand, the risk of an adverse outcome differs considerably, depending on the primary diagnosis. When intervention is not urgent, some delays in prescribing an antibiotic may not increase the risk to the patient and might substantially decrease the use of antibiotics (Edwards, Dennison et al. 2003).

Unfortunately, without a confirmed diagnosis, the doctor must choose among several antibiotics and logically goes with her best bet—a broad-spectrum antibiotic, one that covers the broadest possible range of infecting agents, rather than an antibiotic that targets only a few. Often patients continue a course of antibiotics even after a microbiological test fails to find a bacterial infection. If a bacterial infection is confirmed and the patient is responding to treatment with the initial antibiotic, the doctor is generally reluctant to switch to a narrow-spectrum drug that might have been more appropriate in the first place. (Chapter 3 explores the issue of overprescribing in greater depth.)

A specimen is sometimes sent to the clinic's microbiology laboratory. Lab work becomes extremely valuable if a patient fails to respond to treatment, but treatment failure is uncommon and lab work has a tangible cost. If a microbiological sample was not taken initially, further waiting is required, and this can put patients at further risk.

A microbiological lab report about an antibiotic generally includes the species of bacteria that are present in an infection and a profile of the resistance patterns. These microbiological patterns also form the basis for much of the existing surveillance data. Importantly, the definition of antibiotic resistance from microbiological tests (i.e., *in vitro*) does not always correspond to the results of treatment (i.e., *in vivo*).

These differences affect the ability of doctors to appropriately treat patients and may introduce a major source of bias in all the passive reporting on the frequency of resistance.

Antibiotic therapy can fail for reasons that have nothing to do with evolved resistance. Many bacteria species are intrinsically resistant to antibiotics: some antibiotics are effective against only Gram-positive or only Gram-negative bacteria, some work only on certain species. Bacteria can acquire phenotypic resistance, a kind of acquired resistance that arises in response to antibiotics and is not inherited (Levin 2004; Wiuff, Zappala et al. 2005). Bacteria in biofilms (Box 2.3), which form on medical devices and human tissues, can become persistent sources of infection that are not easy to eliminate or cure (Rotun, McMath et al. 1999). Thus, the evolution of resistance is one of many causes of treatment failure.

■ _____

## Origins of resistant bacteria

Evolved resistance is of greatest interest to policymakers because it is responsible for the increase in the frequency of resistance and because it holds the promise of being managed through policy mechanisms. In practice, policy approaches have met with varying degrees of success. Some bacteria evolve resistance to antibiotics immediately; other species wait decades before resistance emerges, and the reasons for this difference are not well understood. Here, we consider origins and spread as different and important steps in the evolution of resistance. First, we consider the origins of resistance, because the genetic origins of resistance may affect the choice of policy (for a longer discussion of this subject, see Lipsitch and Samore 2002).

Resistant bacteria can evolve *de novo* from a population that was sensitive before treatment in two ways: quantitative changes in resistance through the accumulation of random mutations, and the transfer of whole genes or sets of genes from other bacteria species (Davies 1994). In the first way,

populations can evolve gradually and quantitatively through simple point mutations, which are one-letter changes in the genetic code, or through more significant mutations, such as insertions or deletions in several letters that are mistakenly omitted or copied from somewhere else. This is how other pathogens commonly evolve resistance. In the second way, the potential to acquire whole sets of genes from other species distinguishes bacteria from viruses or eukaryotic pathogens.[2] Either way, for bacteria to become viable and epidemiologically important, further genetic changes may be required after transmission among several hosts and repeated exposure to antibiotics. The evolution of resistance *de novo* refers to the process of selection within a host that transforms a population of sensitive bacteria with a few resistant mutants into a daughter population of bacteria that are efficiently transmitted and dominated by resistant mutants.

Incremental changes in resistance have been understood since antibiotic resistance was discovered. Large phenotypic changes from small genetic changes are possible, but point mutations typically provide small advantages by themselves. Thus, bacteria must accumulate many small mutations to tolerate the high concentrations of drugs given to patients. Steady, incremental increases over time in bacteria's ability to tolerate drugs can be countered by steady increases in the dose of a drug until the toxicity of the drug at high concentrations becomes a problem.

If patients do not comply with a drug regimen, some bacteria survive that are more resistant. These partially sensitive

_____

2  Broadly speaking, pathogens are classified as bacteria, eukaryotes, or viruses. Eukaryotic pathogens, including fungi, various types of intestinal worms, and *Plasmodium falciparum* (the parasite that causes malaria), have a nucleus, they are diploid, and they reproduce sexually. Viruses are bits of genetic material encapsulated in a protein coat, and by most criteria, they are not considered to be alive. Some viruses are composed of several pieces, so it is possible for the genetic material to recombine; influenza is a notable example. Compared with most eukaryotes and viruses, bacteria are extremely promiscuous—they have sex in more ways and with a broader diversity of organisms.

BOX 2.6

## THE BIOLOGICAL COST OF RESISTANCE

The emergence and spread of resistance tend to be slowed because resistant pathogens tend to be less fit than their drug-sensitive relatives, often because the mechanism of resistance interferes with other metabolic pathways. The biological cost of resistance is a fitness cost that may manifest itself as a lower growth rate, higher death rate, or some other competitive disadvantage within a host, as faster clearance from hosts, or as slower transmission rates among hosts. These fitness costs would also cause the decline of resistance in the absence of drug pressure, although the rate of decline might be slower than the rate of increase (Andersson and Levin 1999; Bjorkman and Andersson 2000; Andersson 2006).

Because the biological cost of resistance affects the relationship between antibiotic use and antibiotic resistance, it is an important concept for any policy. In fact, there have been examples of evolved resistance without a biological cost, but a biological cost has been documented for most antibiotic-resistant microbes, whenever it was studied. More commonly, the biological cost declines over time as other mutations arise that compensate for the biological cost (Levin, Perrot et al. 2000; Andersson 2006), so the fitness of drug-resistant bacteria tends to increase until it is not substantially lower than that of the drug-sensitive bacteria.

bacteria spread and mutate, and resistance can increase on further exposure to antibiotics. The solution has been to ensure that patients take a sufficiently massive dose of a drug to completely eliminate the pathogen. Thus, to discourage the rapid evolution of quantitative resistance, emphasis has been placed on compliance with antibiotic treatment, and this has led to the perspective that the evolution of resistance in bacteria is largely an issue of the abuse of antibiotics, including patients' noncompliance and physicians' overprescription.

That point of view, at least with respect to noncompliance with antibiotic drug regimens and the origins of resistance, is not entirely correct, since resistance can emerge by the acquisition of whole genes on genetic elements that are transferred among bacteria, including multiple-drug resistance that is transferred all at once. Many bacteria share genetic material with other closely related and sometimes more distantly related bacteria. In this way, whole genes or sets of genes that work together can move out of one ecological reservoir, such as a soil microbe or farm animal communities, and into another, such as hospital-acquired pathogens. This has been an important way for antibiotic resistance to develop and spread, especially in the case of vancomycin-resistant enterococci (VRE) and methicillin-resistant *S. aureus* (MRSA) and pneumococci (Lipsitch and Samore 2002). Thus, the spread of resistance genes, and not necessarily of bacteria, can be one underlying cause of an epidemic of resistance. Moreover, genes that confer resistance to antibiotics can move around together to provide bacteria with an easy way of becoming resistant to many antibiotics all at once.

Implementing a policy of increasing compliance to discourage the origins of resistance may or may not delay the emergence of resistance, depending on the underlying genetic mechanism. For resistance that is transmitted on mobile genetic elements, compliance is not likely to be effective in delaying the emergence of resistance, and the increased length of compliant treatment prolongs the period of increased risk of colonization by resistant bacteria. In some cases, increased compliance may be counterproductive (Lipsitch and Samore 2002).

## Spread of resistant bacteria

Despite the interest in the emergence of antibiotic resistance, the problem is largely the spread of resistant bacteria or resistance genes, not the repeated evolution of resistance *de novo* (Box 2.5, see next page). Indeed, the spread of a resistant bacterial clone or resistance genes is probably responsible for more clinical failure than *de novo* resistance within a host, so controlling spread should be given much greater concern and attention. In fact, policy should be chosen based on the propensity for resistant bacteria to evolve *de novo* in response to antibiotic use, or to spread. These propensities differ among bacteria species, so different policy solutions may be required for different bacteria.

Why do antibiotic-resistant bacteria spread? This question is, perhaps, wrong minded. Since all bacteria spread, given the opportunity, why would antibiotic-resistant bacteria *not* spread? Not all bacteria are successful; ultimately, bacteria are limited by many other factors, including other bacteria. In the intensely competitive microbial world, resistant bacteria are thought to be at an inherent disadvantage because of the biological cost of resistance (Box 2.6). The weight of evidence supporting a biological cost of resistance includes some strong *a priori* reasoning, in addition to direct observational and experimental evidence (Andersson and Levin 1999). The biological costs may be manifest as slower growth rates within a host that would make resistant bacteria lose out in head-to-head competition with other bacteria. Resistant bacteria may be shed at lower rates and spread less efficiently, or they may clear faster, thus providing fewer opportunities to spread. Evidence also suggests that the biological cost of resistance

is highest just after resistance evolves, and then declines over time as compensatory mutations arise that reduce the biological cost of resistance (Levin, Perrot et al. 2000).

Countering the biological cost of resistance, the use of antibiotics in a bacteria population confers two main fitness advantages to the resistant bacteria. First, the use of antibiotics reduces the fitness of sensitive bacteria by increasing their clearance rates. Second, as the concentrations of antibiotic wane, resistant bacteria have a window of opportunity when they can colonize a host but sensitive bacteria cannot. When these fitness advantages are strong enough to compensate for the biological cost of resistance (see Box 2.6), resistant bacteria tend to spread.

Put another way, the use of antibiotics shifts the balance in favor of resistant bacteria over sensitive bacteria, and the among-host fitness advantages created by antibiotic use outweigh the biological cost of resistance. When these ideas are encapsulated into a mathematical model, a simple principle arises: there are thresholds on the rate of antibiotic use that favor resistant bacteria (Austin, Kristinsson et al.

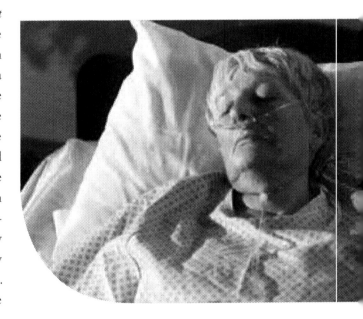

BOX 2.5

# THE RELATIONSHIP BETWEEN ANTIBIOTIC USE AND ANTIBIOTIC RESISTANCE

The rising frequency of antibiotic resistance is obviously due to antibiotic use, but what is the relationship between antibiotic use and antibiotic resistance? Antibiotic use can select for resistance within a host, so any direct comparison of bacteria can find higher levels of resistance after chemotherapy (e.g., see Dowell and Schwartz 1997), but this is only one possible explanation for the rising frequency of resistance. Such patterns may differ, depending on the particular microbe and antibiotic considered. The alternative explanation is that antibiotic-resistant bacteria tend to spread once they have evolved, especially in populations where antibiotic use is heavy.

To understand the spread of antibiotic-resistant bacteria (or resistance genes), it is necessary to understand both transmission and persistence. Resistance tends to a steady state when the number of people who are newly colonized equals the number of people in whom resistant bacteria are eliminated. A clone will tend to persist in a population of hosts if, when almost no other host is colonized, it spreads faster than it clears. Thus, the steady state can be lowered by slowing transmission rates or increasing clearance rates, and if either one of these interventions reduces the steady state below a threshold, the clone will be eliminated.

Antibiotic-resistant bacteria are like other pathogens: to establish themselves in a population, they must be able to colonize new hosts faster than they are cleared. They differ from other pathogens in one important way: they share the same niche with drug-sensitive bacteria (e.g., Dall'Antonia, Coen et al. 2005). In other words, both resistant and sensitive bacteria inhibit each other. Thus, antibiotic-resistant bacteria must be able to increase when they are rare, despite colonization inhibition from their drug-sensitive competitors. To understand the spread of resistance, it is therefore necessary to first understand the spread of the species overall, and then to look at the relative dynamics of the resistant and sensitive bacteria together.

Epidemiological models (Box 2.2) suggest that resistance will tend to increase in frequency if resistant bacteria are more fit than their drug-sensitive relatives. In this context, fitness is measured in terms of the number of new hosts colonized, the product of the number of contacts per day, and the average number of days that shedding continues before the bacteria clear. In simple models (e.g., Bonhoeffer, Lipsitch et al. 1997), antibiotic use increases the clearance rates of drug-sensitive pathogens. On the other hand, antibiotic-resistant bacteria may spread less efficiently or be eliminated faster because of the biological cost of resistance (Box 2.6). At some frequency of antibiotic use, clearance of drug-sensitive pathogens is increased sufficiently by antibiotic use to shift the competitive balance in favor of resistant pathogens. Since the rate of antibiotic use is related to the lower fitness of sensitive bacteria, there is a threshold on selection that determines when resistance will tend to increase. The selection threshold describes a drug prescription rate that exactly balances the biological cost of resistance. Below the threshold, resistant bacteria would not increase in frequency because of competitive inhibition with drug-sensitive bacteria. Above the threshold, resistant bacteria can increase in frequency despite ongoing competition.

This sort of analysis suggests that the spread of resistance depends on the level of antibiotic use within a population, not on antibiotic use by individuals. Resistance tends to increase in a population wherever the selective balance is tipped, so the increase in resistance within a population would be related to total antibiotic use, not necessarily by any one individual's antibiotic use (Lipsitch, Bergstrom et al. 2000). For antibiotic resistance, causation must be investigated by comparing populations that differ in their level of antibiotic use, or by comparing the relationship between variance in antibiotic use and antibiotic resistance in a single population over time (Monnet and Lopez-Lozano 2005).

Antibiotic use by individuals might increase their personal risk of carrying some antibiotic-resistant pathogens, but because of spread, the risk of carrying resistance would be most closely related to measures of exposure, such as recent hospitalization, not personal antibiotic use (Lipsitch 2001; Carmeli, Eliopoulos et al. 2002). Methods developed to investigate causation for cancer and heart disease focus on individual-level causes, so they may be misleading when applied to group-level causation, such as the relationship between antibiotic use and antibiotic resistance; the lack of an association between an individual's history of antibiotic use and antibiotic resistance does not mean that antibiotic use is not the cause of antibiotic resistance, just that it may not be an individual-level cause. There are, moreover, two relevant ways of measuring risk: an individual's risk of carrying some resistant bacteria, and an individual's likelihood of carrying drug-resistant bacteria rather than their drug-sensitive competitor. The second measure of risk is problematic because antibiotics would clear sensitive bacteria and thus increase the risk of carrying resistance, but not because it actually increased colonization with resistant bacteria (Lipsitch 2001).

In sum, theory suggests that there is some threshold on antibiotic use; below that threshold, resistance would be unable to persist. It may be possible to control the spread of resistant pathogens through some combination of strategies that limits the resistant pathogen more than its competitors. The main ways to do this are by limiting antibiotic use and by improving infection control. To be effective against resistance, infection control must be applied more aggressively against resistant pathogens. Without differential application of infection control, transmission is reduced for both resistant and sensitive pathogens, but there is no net selective pressure to counter the effects of selection by antibiotics.

Another important concern is that after stopping all antibiotic use, antibiotic resistance is expected to decline much more slowly than it increased (Bonhoeffer, Lipsitch et al. 1997). As a consequence, strategies that slow the increase, such as using several antibiotics simultaneously to reduce selection by all of them, would tend to be much more effective than strategies that rest antibiotics by stopping use, such as cycling (Bonhoeffer, Lipsitch et al. 1997; Bergstrom, Lo et al. 2004).

Given the differences in the bacteria and the antibiotics, it is most likely that no single rule of thumb can be applied to every situation. One of the most important aims of basic research should be to describe the range of possible outcomes, and a set of policy options that are suitable for a particular drug-bug combination.

1999). If the rate of use is below the threshold, the frequency of resistance tends to decline. If the rate of use is high enough, resistant bacteria increase in frequency. Thus, an important factor is the rate that an antibiotic is used in a population.

The rate of antibiotic use is too low in most places to favor resistance, but antibiotics are heavily used in hospitals and other health care facilities. These institutions are connected by repeated hospitalization and the transfer of patients to and from hospitals and long-term care facilities (Smith, Dushoff et al. 2004). This leads to a view of the resistance epidemic that focuses on controlling transmission of resistant bacteria in places where antibiotic use is heaviest (HICPAC 1995; Weinstein 2001). Hospitals and long-term care facilities (Nicolle 2001; Elizaga, Weinstein et al. 2002) are regarded as "sources" because a greater fraction of patients leave a hospital colonized with resistant bacteria than entered, and

the surrounding community is a "sink" where the frequency of colonization tends to decrease. The declining resistance in sinks is due to natural turnover and the clearance of resistant pathogens and low transmission rates. Thus, at least some part of the public health response should be to identify and focus control efforts on those institutions that are sources—usually places where antibiotics are heavily used (Hartley, Furuno et al. 2006). Important source institutions are hospitals, long-term care facilities, daycare centers, and prisons.

The source-sink dynamic interacts with underlying heterogeneity in the human population, and some subpopulations probably play a particularly important role in the spread of antibiotic resistance. One class of important players is health care workers, who are in the hospital every day (Trick, Weinstein et al. 2001). Since resistant bacteria can be extremely persistent, patients who are frequently

BOX 2.7

## VANCOMYCIN-RESISTANT ENTEROCOCCI

Enterococci are not generally pathogenic—they colonize the gut during the first few days of life, for example—and fecal-to-oral transmission of enterococci is common. Most infections are hospital acquired. Serious infections with enterococci are most common in the urinary tract and the intra-abdominal cavity, and IV- and catheter-associated infections often arise in critically ill patients. Endocarditis is a common and dangerous complication of enterococcal bacteremia. Enterococci were long regarded as harmless gut commensals that caused mild infections until most acquired resistance to aminoglycosides and then vancomycin in 1987 (Rice 2001). In the late 1980s and early 1990s, VRE spread rapidly within U.S. and European hospitals. The bacteria were then heralded as a "superbug" because they were not treatable by any approved antibiotics until 1999–2000, when two new antibiotics were approved for VRE, MRSA, and other Gram-positive bacteria: synercid (quinupristin and dalfopristin) and linezolid. The long history of avoparcin use in many European countries in agriculture for growth promotion sparked a controversy about the origins of vancomycin resistance and the effects of growth promoters (Bonten, Willems et al. 2001).

hospitalized or who have very long hospital visits likely play an important role in the establishment of endemic populations (Furuno, McGregor et al. 2006).

In addition to health care workers and patients, the institution itself—the building, furniture, and equipment—can become contaminated with antibiotic-resistant bacteria, especially species that are able to persist for long periods in the environment. Some species of bacteria are very durable and can persist on bed frames, couches, medical instruments, and other objects, from which they can continue to contaminate the hands of health care workers and patients. Such contamination may play an important role in the establishment of endemic populations of resistance in hospitals and long-term care facilities (Hayden, Bonten et al. 2006).

Importantly, few antibiotics are used for just one bacterial pathogen, and few bacteria are resistant to just one antibiotic, but most studies of antibiotic resistance have focused on the "one-bug, one-drug" problem. Another conceptual model for the emergence of resistance is that antibiotic use has acted as a major perturbation to microbial communities, and that the emergence of resistance is the result of disturbing whole communities. In these disturbed environments, the bacteria that have thrived are those that are naturally invasive—the equivalent of weeds. This may account for the emergence of enterococci and VRE as important hospital-acquired infections in the 1980s (Box 2.7). Long-term changes in the frequency of *Enterococcus faecalis* and *E. faecium* and the increased frequency of *Clostridium difficile* infections may be important medical side effects of community-level changes that are driven by antibiotic use.

There are, of course, other ways that resistance can spread rapidly through a population. One is the accidental spread by hitchhiking on other successful genes. Since resistance genes are all likely to be successful in the same places, several antibiotic resistance genes can all travel together on the same mobile genetic element and contribute to the increasing frequency of bacteria that are resistant to more than one antibiotic. Another way is for resistance to be present in the founding member of a very successful clone; such founder effects may account for recent changes in the epidemiology of MRSA (Box 2.8). Since genes move among bacteria, some bacteria species that are not important pathogens are nevertheless clinically important because they act as a reservoir of resistance genes. The relative importance of all these mechanisms has not been fully explored.

## The aim of control

When considering the control of antibiotic-resistant bacteria, what should be the goal? Given the complex biology and epidemiology of antibiotic resistance, there are several possible goals. One is to delay the emergence of antibiotic resistance. Another is to slow the spread with the long-term goal of reducing the frequency of resistance, or at least reducing the rate at which the frequency is increasing. A third goal is to reduce the number of infections with antibiotic-resistant bacteria. These goals often point to the same interventions for controlling resistant infections, but not always.

Reducing the frequency of resistance is not, in and of itself, the primary goal of policy. If all one wanted to do was reverse the spread of resistance, one could simply stop using all antibiotics. If no antibiotic resistance had emerged, newly evolved strains would certainly not have an advantage, so the frequency of antibiotic resistance would decline, albeit slowly, because of the biological cost of resistance. Antibiotics are valuable, however, because of their ability to treat infections. Although eliminating antibiotic use may be effective in minimizing resistance, this would be like never driving one's car to avoid scratching it.

On the other hand, one could simply prevent as many infections as possible, but since some infection is inevitable, preventing infections is only a partially effective goal. If a policy does not reverse an increasing trend in the frequency of resistance, eventually all the infections will be resistant.

What is the right goal for a program to control antibiotic resistance? If we consider antibiotic effectiveness a scarce resource, the obvious goal is to maximize the total net benefit of an antibiotic in a population over time. The total benefit should be weighted toward treating people who are sick in the present and people with a critical need in the future, rather than people who might receive a marginal benefit in the present. The preference for discounting future resistance has a medical justification, in addition to the economic reasons for discounting the future. New therapies to treat infections may be available in the future that are not available today, so future infections are always discounted by the expectation that they will be treatable by other means.

The goal of maximizing the total net benefit of an antibiotic can be accomplished by delaying the emergence of resistance, by slowing the spread of resistance to reduce the frequency of antibiotic-resistant infections, and by reducing the total number of infections. To find the balance of strategies that would maximize the right objective function, some new analysis is required.

■
_____

## Controlling antibiotic use

The best and most obvious way to delay emergence and slow spread is to reduce selection by eliminating the use of antibiotics when they do not provide any medical benefit. Doctors often prescribe antibiotics unnecessarily for several reasons: 1) the patient and doctor have a different incentive to treat an infection than society; 2) there is always some uncertainty associated with diagnosing a medical problem; 3) reducing that uncertainty requires time and money; 4) all else equal, antibiotics are most likely to benefit a patient if the treatment is started early; and 5) patients want antibiotics

when they are not needed, for various reasons (see Chapter 3 on patient and physician demand for antibiotics).

To put it another way, what happens when a patient presents with symptoms that are occasionally caused by bacteria but usually caused by something else? The doctor can either prescribe empiric therapy or wait until a diagnostic test confirms a bacterial infection. The decision to use an antibiotic immediately gives the patient something tangible to take away from the visit and makes him feel better, protects a doctor's liability on the off-chance that the infection was bacterial, and eliminates the time, expense, and delay of an additional visit and laboratory diagnostic tests. On the other hand, diagnostic tests can help the doctor identify the cause of an infection and, especially in the case of inappropriate empiric therapy, choose more appropriate treatments. Thus, increased use of diagnostic tools can help reduce treatment failures from other causes and reduce mortality (Fagon, Chastre et al. 2000).

Offsetting those incentives and benefits are the cost of the antibiotic, the risk of an adverse reaction to the medicine, and the risk of resistance. All of these costs are mitigated for the doctor and patient: the doctor doesn't pay for the antibiotic and the patient's prescription drugs are often subsidized. Doctors are not typically regarded as liable for adverse reactions, and patients do not regard antibiotics as dangerous. Although the patient does increase his risk of antibiotic resistance in future infections from the increased resistance in his resident flora, that threat seems remote.

Cultural norms and other factors also influence the desire to take antibiotics, but the above caricature of the complex negotiation between doctor and patient illustrates several of the reasons why it is difficult to reduce unnecessary antibiotic use.

One suggestion is that delaying prescriptions for some kinds of infections could reduce antibiotic use without placing patients at elevated risk (Edwards, Dennison et al. 2003).

**BOX 2.8**

## METHICILLIN-RESISTANT *STAPHYLOCOCCUS AUREUS* (MRSA)

*Staphylococcus aureus* colonizes the anterior nares but is also sometimes found colonizing the gut (Kluytmans, Belkam et al. 1997). Despite frequent carriage, it is known as a relatively aggressive and virulent pathogen that causes food poisoning, pneumonia, mastitis, phlebitis, and urinary tract infections, as well as minor infections of the skin. In the most severe cases it can cause osteomyelitis and endocarditis, hospital-acquired infections, infections of surgical wounds, and device-associated infections.

Although oxacillin is now used instead of methicillin, this bacterium is still commonly referred to as MRSA, and it is typically resistant to multiple antibiotics. MRSA now accounts for more than 60 percent of *S. aureus* infections in hospital intensive care units (CDC 2004), which are most often treated with vancomycin. The van genes that confer vancomycin resistance in enterococci have been transferred to MRSA both *in vitro* and *in vivo* (CDC 2002a; CDC 2002b), but so far, high-level vancomycin resistance in MRSA has not spread. Nevertheless, there is fear that vancomycin resistance will emerge and begin to spread.

In the early 1990s MRSA was principally associated with hospital-acquired infections, but in the mid-1990s the epidemiology of MRSA began to change because of the spread of a new pandemic clone with a new staphylococcal chromosomal cassette type (Herold, Immergluck et al. 1998; Kluytmans-Vandenbergh and Kluytmans 2006). Now, the two main types of MRSA are hospital acquired (HA-MRSA) and community acquired (CA-MRSA), although MRSA strains that are typically community acquired are occasionally acquired in a hospital and vice versa. CA-MRSA infections are more virulent (i.e. colonization is much more likely to result in an infection), but typically milder than HA-MRSA infections, largely because of factors related to the host. CA-MRSA is often associated with skin infections, but they can also be very severe. Recent epidemics of CA-MRSA have occurred in prisons, the military, and other populations (CDC 2003; Aiello, Lowy et al. 2006). As CA-MRSA has spread, the epidemiology of HA-MRSA and CA-MRSA has become increasingly similar.

In addition to *S. aureus*, around 80 percent of infections with coagulase-negative *Staphylococcus* spp. are resistant to beta-lactams, and 80 percent are methicillin resistant. These staphylococcal species include *S. epidermis*.

Another way to reduce the total selective pressure applied by today's drugs is to shift away from broad-spectrum antibiotics to narrow-spectrum antibiotics. A broad-spectrum antibiotic is more likely to work against an infection with unidentified bacteria. Despite the advantages to the patient, the broad-spectrum antibiotic selects for resistance in several bacteria species all at once. A narrow-spectrum antibiotic should limit the collateral damage. Unfortunately, there is not much research to support these assertions, since the effects of various antibiotics on the emergence of resistance within multiple species have not been studied.

Unnecessary antibiotic use and a shift from broad- to narrow-spectrum antibiotics would be facilitated if rapid diagnostic tests were available and affordable, and if the financial incentives to doctors and patients were changed to encourage their use. However, many bacteria that cause infections are not easily cultured and may not be detected with a rapid diagnostic test. Although some unidentifiable bacterial infections make up a small percentage of infections, they do occur. Rapid diagnostic tests could be improved with new technology, but the rapid tests are neither perfect nor inexpensive, and increasing testing can strain the microbiological resources of a hospital.

Finally, antibiotic resistance may be managed by manipulating the relative amounts of different antibiotics that are used. One proposed strategy is to rotate or cycle antibiotics. Although there are solid a priori arguments in favor of cycling antibiotics, a recent systematic review found insufficient evidence to evaluate cycling as a policy (Masterton 2005). Available ecological theory also suggests that concurrent use of multiple antibiotics would be more effective than cycling (Bonhoeffer, Lipsitch et al. 1997; Bergstrom, Lo et al. 2004), but there is very little high-quality empirical evidence to evaluate these strategies. A closely related strategy that reduces the number of antibiotic-resistant infections is to clear the colonizing bacteria, usually with some other antibiotic; for

## Antibiotics should be taken if there is a danger that a partially treated infection will come back, but what if a patient has started on antibiotics and a subsequent diagnostic test reveals that the infection is not bacterial?

example, mupirocin is often used to eliminate colonization with MRSA in patients who are at risk of infection (Perl, Cullen et al. 2002). This is a useful strategy, but resistance to the alternative antibiotic is also a concern.

A controversial bit of advice that does not unambiguously stem the rising tide of antibiotics is to "take the full course of antibiotics." Antibiotics should be taken if there is a danger that a partially treated infection will recrudesce, but what if a patient has started on antibiotics and a subsequent diagnostic test reveals that the infection is not bacterial? Should he continue to take a full course of antibiotics? At its extreme, the full course of antibiotics increases the total amount of antibiotics used and increases the possibilities for collateral damage. This advice clearly needs a more critical evaluation.

That raises the closely related issue of the design of antibiotic courses in general. Is the duration of a course of antibiotics longer than it needs to be to clear an infection? Once the risk of recrudescence has passed, so has the need for antibiotics, but continued use may contribute to the spread of resistance. Improving antibiotic dosing by taking short, intense courses could be an important part of limiting antibiotic use, but it would require substantial additional PK/PD research (for example, see Schrag et al. 2001). This suggests that antibiotics should be given more intensively and for shorter intervals, a general principle that is finding increasing application (Drusano 2003; Drusano 2005).

■
_____

## Controlling infection

Another strategy for controlling resistance is to reduce transmission of bacteria. Indeed, the Hospital Infection Control Practices Advisory Committee recommendations for controlling VRE include advice about reducing transmission of these pathogens from patient to patient (HICPAC 1995). Hospital infection control has at least two important goals, one of which is to protect individual patients from infections. This would presumably limit opportunities for the spread of VRE and eliminate outbreaks. A secondary effect may be to reduce the number of bacterial infections, and thus reduce the total amount of antibiotics used.

The other purpose of hospital infection control, one that is identified for the first time in this report, is to reduce the fitness of antibiotic-resistant bacteria. From the perspective of an individual human host, there are two ways to manipulate the among-host component of bacterial fitness: slow transmission or reduce persistence. An important principle is that antibiotic resistance can be controlled without eliminating all antibiotic use or completely isolating every patient. Antibiotic-resistant pathogens can be thought of in two ways, for the purposes of control: they can be considered a simple pathogen, or they can be considered competition for drug-sensitive bacteria. Either way, controlling the spread of resistance involves threshold phenomena: it is sufficient to reduce the rate of transmission such that every pathogen is spread from each person to less than one other person, or that the resistant strains spread less efficiently than sensitive strains.

That evolutionary perspective is critical. Any action taken to reduce transmission in some general way reduces transmission for drug-sensitive bacteria as well. Thus, to be most effective, hospital infection control should be applied selectively—that is, it should be applied more strenuously and effectively against resistant bacteria. In other words, the best hospital infection control policy is to be selectively clean.

What are the most effective ways to slow transmission? Since health care workers act as vectors that carry resistant bacteria among patients, via contaminated hands, clothing, or medical instruments, simple measures to reduce transmission include hand washing, gloves, gowns, and other barrier precautions. Other strategies include more careful decontamination of medical instruments and having health care workers trim their fingernails and remove neckties. Transmission can also be improved by limiting the number of contacts: isolating colonized or at-risk patients, reducing nurses' workloads, or decreasing cohorting (i.e., reducing the number of patients seen by each nurse).

Another effective way of reducing resistance is to eliminate the resistant bacteria that have colonized the hospital environment. Some kinds of bacteria are extremely durable and persist on hospital equipment for weeks or months. The frequency of resistance can be reduced by improving cleaning procedures (Hayden, Bonten et al. 2006). Health care workers who may be carriers of resistance are yet another target (Lessing, Jordens et al. 1996; Lange, Morrissey et al. 2000; Trick, Weinstein et al. 2001; Baran, Ramanathan et al. 2002).

Some hospital infection control measures have been difficult to implement or sustain, however. Improved hand washing is typically difficult to achieve unless hospitals make dramatic changes, such as altering hospital architecture to make hand-washing sinks readily available, or including hand washing as a performance measure linked to pay and promotion. Such practices would need to be enforced on doctors as well as nurses.

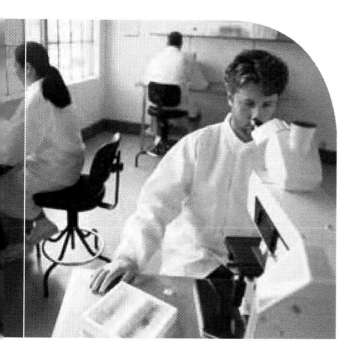

about the antibiotic-resistant bacteria that are known to colonize a patient. The development of a personal electronic medical history that includes laboratory test results, previous antibiotics used, and other information would make this strategy efficient and offer other benefits, such as providing doctors with a more complete patient history. The record could be useful for hospitals to identify and isolate potential carriers.

Fewer options exist for reducing the persistence time of resistant bacteria, except possibly through selective decontamination. Some other interventions may be found through focused research on the ecological relationships among bacteria, which could reduce the prevalence of colonization with medically important species.

## Novel ecological strategies

Ecological strategies might also counter the effects of antibiotic use. If antibiotic resistance has spread because antibiotic use has opened a niche, that niche could be filled with something else. In general, this something else would have to be another bacterial species, one that is not pathogenic. Harmless bacteria that are taken for such purposes are called probiotics. In fact, probiotics are a common part of informal health care: people often eat live-culture yogurt after taking antibiotics to restore their normal flora. Probiotics have a place in treating bacterial overgrowth, but the therapeutic and public health value of probiotics to reduce antibiotic resistance is not well studied, and early results are not promising (Lund, Edlund et al. 2000; Lund, Adamsson et al. 2002).

Another source of resistance is the hospital patients themselves. One of the major problems with hospital infection control is that it fails to identify many patients who are already colonized by antibiotic-resistant bacteria at the time of admission. A solution is to test patients on admission, a process known as active surveillance. It is, of course, expensive to test everyone and isolate patients, but studies suggest it would be cost-effective (Perencevich, Fisman et al. 2004). Patients can be isolated until they return a negative test or isolated after they test positive; the former strategy would be more effective but more expensive. A simple way to reduce the number of patients to be tested while still identifying most carriers is to focus on patients who have significant risk factors, such as having been recently hospitalized (Furuno, McGregor et al. 2006), admitted from a long-term care facility, or prescribed antibiotics.

Given the costs of active surveillance, an alternative strategy would be for hospitals to share information with each other

Another possibility is to exploit biological control agents. For example, a bacteriophage that attacks particular strains of bacteria could be engineered and spread around to decontaminate a hospital or to reduce bacterial colonization of the skin. These strategies are largely speculative.

A successful policy will have a solid epidemiological basis but must also follow economic principles. Since antibiotic resistance spreads among hospitals, states, and nations, any program used by one agent to control the spread of resistance within its own borders can be undermined by the inaction of a neighbor. Players acting in their own self-interest, moreover, may not behave in a way that benefits the common good. Without coordination, some players may choose to free-ride on the investments of their neighbors. For example, hospitals that share patients may choose to free-ride on the infection-control policies of other nearby hospitals (Smith, Levin et al. 2005). When all players adopt that strategy, the result is a Nash equilibrium—a perfectly rational but unfortunate global strategy.

## Success stories

The policies for controlling the spread of resistance in the United States and across the world have largely failed, but a few success stories do exist. Two are the Dutch experience with MRSA control, and VRE control in the Siouxland (also discussed in Chapter 4). Both of these approaches were very aggressive, and both involved coordination at some large regional level.

In the Netherlands, patients admitted to hospitals from outside the country were automatically quarantined. When transmission did occur, radical measures were taken to control transmission; when transmission was documented, hospital units were shut down. Dutch citizens were not tracked individually, but they were known to be safe because the national policy was universally followed and MRSA was so rare. A few expensive outbreaks of MRSA were identified with Dutch citizens who became carriers while hospitalized outside the Dutch system (Verhoef, Beaujean et al. 1999). Despite the inconvenience and the huge expense of the "search-and-destroy" strategy, it was cost-effective because it reduced the number of infections of both VRE and MRSA (Vriens, Blok et al. 2002).

One notable effect of the Dutch strategy was to reduce transmission of *S. aureus* and select against the most transmissible clone until it was eliminated from the Netherlands (Verhoef, Beaujean et al. 1999). Thus, as time went on, hospital infection control measures had the added benefit of selecting for bacterial pathogens that were easier to control.

In Siouxland—where Iowa, Nebraska, and South Dakota meet—several hospitals coordinated their efforts. They tracked patients who had become carriers and quarantined them when they entered other hospitals. This strategy, combined with patient isolation measures, led to decreases in the transmission and prevalence of VRE (Ostrowsky, Trick et al. 2001; Sohn, Ostrowsky et al. 2001).

Major shifts in the epidemiology of disease have been caused by the evolution of pathogens unrelated to resistance, and these should be regarded as important side effects—both positive and negative—of the use of antibiotics and of enlightened infection control. As mentioned, the radical hospital infection control procedures in the Netherlands eliminated one of the most transmissible types of *S. aureus*. And acute rheumatic fever is now rare in the United States, mostly because of treatment of Group A streptococcal infections with penicillin (Krause 2002). An increasing incidence of *Clostridium difficile* infections, however, may be a negative side effect of antibiotic use.

## Summary

The spread of resistance is an ecological problem involving competition between sensitive and resistant bacteria. Resistant bacteria may have inherent disadvantages or fitness costs when they first evolve, but these disadvantages may evolve away over time. Antibiotic-resistant bacteria are infectious agents, and the conditions for spread involve thresholds. Because of these thresholds and the complex ecology of resistant bacteria, the design and control of antibiotic resistance are difficult to study, and interpretation of data is often not straightforward (Lipsitch, Bergstrom et al. 2000). The success of various control measures may not become apparent unless they reduce selection below a threshold, and the effects may not become apparent until the ecological reservoir of resistance is reduced—a process that could take years.

There are real obstacles to changing the way antibiotics are used, and real difficulties in slowing the spread of resistance. Coordination and investment have been insufficient. Many potential solutions to the problem of resistance exist, but the incentives of the agents are not aligned, and it is unlikely that any of these solutions will work without structural changes to the way all the agents deal with antibiotic resistance. Cooperation among institutions is difficult, and active surveillance to identify carriers who are entering an institution is expensive for single hospitals. Despite all this, there have been some successes when efforts were coordinated across wide regions. Electronic records, combined with screening algorithms on admission to recognize potential carriers, would improve coordination and have other benefits as well. Most of these problems and potential solutions are dealt with in greater detail in other chapters.

The real costs and benefits of various control measures have not been properly quantified in a controlled environment. Further study and concerted efforts to implement policy measures at scale are necessary to deal with the problem of antibiotic resistance.

## RESEARCH QUESTIONS

**1.** What nonpathogenic bacteria species (or coalitions of species) inhibit colonization by species that are pathogenic or occasionally pathogenic?

**2.** What are the population-level benefits of reducing antibiotic use?

**3.** Does increased compliance with long antibiotic courses encourage the spread of resistance?

**4.** Do rapid diagnostic tests really improve antibiotic use?

**5.** Can antibiotics be used more optimally—for example, through control of hospital formularies—to extend their useful therapeutic life?

**6.** How can hospital infection control and vaccines (i.e., to limit demand for antibiotics) be used to manage resistance?

# References

Agvald-Ohman, C., B. Lund, et al. (2004). "Multiresistant Coagulase-Negative Staphylococci Disseminate Frequently Between Intubated Patients in a Multidisciplinary Intensive Care Unit." *Critical Care* 8(1): 42-47.

Aiello, A. E., F. D. Lowy, et al. (2006). "Meticillin-Resistant *Staphylococcus aureus* Among US Prisoners and Military Personnel: Review and Recommendations for Future Studies." *Lancet Infectious Diseases* 6(6): 335-341.

Andersson, D. I. (2006). "The Biological Cost of Mutational Antibiotic Resistance: Any Practical Conclusions?" *Current Opinion Microbiology* 9(5): 461-5.

Andersson, D. I. and B. R. Levin. (1999). "The Biological Cost of Antibiotic Resistance." *Current Opinion in Microbiology* 2(5): 489-493.

Antia, R., R. R. Regoes, et al. (2003). "The Role of Evolution in the Emergence of Infectious Diseases." *Nature* 426(6967): 658-661.

Aubry-Damon, H., K. Grenet, et al. (2004). "Antimicrobial Resistance in Commensal Flora of Pig Farmers." *Emerging Infectious Diseases* 10(5): 873-879.

Austin, D. J., M. Kakehashi, et al. (1997). "The Transmission Dynamics of Antibiotic-Resistant Bacteria: The Relationship Between Resistance in Commensal Organisms and Antibiotic Consumption." *Proceedings of the Royal Society of London*. Series B 264: 1629-1638.

Austin, D. J., K. G. Kristinsson, et al. (1999). "The Relationship Between the Volume of Antimicrobial Consumption in Human Communities and the Frequency of Resistance." *Proceedings of the National Academy of Sciences of the United States of America* 96: 1152-1156.

Baran, J., J. Ramanathan, et al. (2002). "Stool Colonization with Vancomycin-Resistant Enterococci in Health care Workers and their Households." *Infection Control and Hospital Epidemiology* 23: 23-26.

Becker, N. (1989). *Analysis of Infectious Disease Data*. London: Chapman and Hall.

Bergstrom, C. T., M. Lo, et al. (2004). "Ecological Theory Suggests that Antimicrobial Cycling Will Not Reduce Antimicrobial Resistance in Hospitals." *Proceedings of the National Academy of Sciences of the United States of America* 101: 13285-13290.

Bjorkman, J. and D. I. Andersson. (2000). "The Cost of Antibiotic Resistance from a Bacterial Perspective." *Drug Resistance Updates* 3(4): 237-245.

Bonhoeffer, S., M. Lipsitch, et al. (1997). "Evaluating Treatment Protocols to Prevent Antibiotic Resistance." *Proceedings of the National Academy of Sciences of the United States of America* 94: 12106-12111.

Bonten, M. J., M. K. Hayden, et al. (1996). "Epidemiology of Colonisation of Patients and Environment with Vancomycin-Resistant Enterococci." *Lancet* 348: 1615-1619.

Bonten, M. J., S. Slaughter, et al. (1998). "The Role of Colonization Pressure in the Spread of Vancomycin-Resistant Enterococci: An Important Infection Control Variable." *Archives of Internal Medicine* 158: 1127-1132.

Bonten, M. J., R. Willems, et al. (2001). "Vancomycin-Resistant Enterococci: Why Are They Here, and Where Do They Come From?" *The Lancet Infectious Diseases* 1: 314-325.

Carbon, C. (1999). "Costs of Treating Infections Caused by Methicillin-Resistant Staphylococci and Vancomycin-Resistant Enterococci." *The Journal of Antimicrobial Chemotherapy* 44(Suppl A): 31-36.

Carmeli, Y., G. M. Eliopoulos, et al. (2002). "Antecedent Treatment with Different Antibiotic Agents as a Risk Factor for Vancomycin-Resistant Enterococcus." *Emerging Infectious Diseases* 8(8): 802-7.

CDC. (2002a). "*Staphylococcus aureus* Resistant to Vancomycin—United States, 2002." *MMWR. Morbidity and Mortality Weekly Report* 51: 565-567. Centers for Disease Control and Prevention.

———. (2002b). "Public Health Dispatch: Vancomycin-Resistant *Staphylococcus aureus*—Pennsylvania, 2002." *MMWR. Morbidity and Mortality Weekly Report* 51: 902.

———. (2003). "Methicillin-Resistant *Staphylococcus aureus* Infections in Correctional Facilities—Georgia, California, and Texas, 2001-2003." *MMWR. Morbidity and Mortality Weekly Report* 52(41): 992-996.

———. (2004). "National Nosocomial Infections Surveillance (NNIS) System Report, Data Summary from January 1992 Through June 2004, Issued October 2004." *American Journal of Infection Control* 32: 470-485.

Cooper, B. S., G. F. Medley, et al. (1999). "Preliminary Analysis of the Transmission Dynamics of Nosocomial Infections: Stochastic and Management Effects." *The Journal of Hospital Infection* 43: 131-147.

Cooper, B. S., G. F. Medley, et al. (2004). "Methicillin-Resistant *Staphylococcus aureus* in Hospitals and the Community: Stealth Dynamics and Control Catastrophes." *Proceedings of the National Academy of Sciences of the United States of America* 101: 10223-10228.

Costerton, J. W., P. S. Stewart, et al. (1999). "Bacterial Biofilms: A Common Cause of Persistent Infections." *Science* 284(5418): 1318-1322.

Courvalin, P. (2000). "Will Avilamycin Convert Ziracine into Zerocine?" *Emerging Infectious Diseases* 6(5): 558.

Dall'Antonia, M., P. G. Coen, et al. (2005). "Competition Between Methicillin-Sensitive and -Resistant *Staphylococcus aureus* in the Anterior Nares." *The Journal of Hospital Infection* 61(1): 62-7.

Davies, J. (1994). "Inactivation of Antibiotics and the Dissemination of Resistance Genes." *Science* 264: 375-382.

Donskey, C. J., T. K. Chowdhry, et al. (2000). "Effect of Antibiotic Therapy on the Density of Vancomycin-Resistant Enterococci in the Stool of Colonized Patients." *The New England Journal of Medicine* 28: 1925-1932.

Donskey, C. J., J. A. Hanrahan, et al. (1999). "Effect of Parenteral Antibiotic Administration on Persistence of Vancomycin-Resistant *Enterococcus faecium* in the Mouse Gastrointestinal Tract." *The Journal of Infectious Diseases* 180: 384-390.

———. (2000). "Effect of Parenteral Antibiotic Administration on the Establishment of Colonization with Vancomycin-Resistant *Enterococcus faecium* in the Mouse Gastrointestinal Tract." *The Journal of Infectious Diseases* 181: 1830-1833.

Dowell, S. F. and B. Schwartz. (1997). "Resistant Pneumococci: Protecting Patients Through Judicious Use of Antibiotics." *American Family Physician* 55(5): 1647-54, 1657-8.

Drusano, G. L. (2003). "Prevention of Resistance: A Goal for Dose Selection for Antimicrobial Agents." *Clinical Infectious Diseases* 36(Suppl 1): 42-50.

———. (2005). "Infection Site Concentrations: Their Therapeutic Importance and the Macrolide and Macrolide-Like Class of Antibiotics." *Pharmacotherapy* 25(12 Pt 2): 150S-158S.

Dykes, G. A. (1995). "Bacteriocins: Ecological and Evolutionary Significance." *Trends in Ecology & Evolution* 10(5): 186-189.

Dykes, G. A. and J. W. Hastings. (1997). "Selection and Fitness in Bacteriocin-Producing Bacteria." *Proceedings of the Royal Society of London*. Series B 264(1382): 683-687.

Edwards, M., J. Dennison, et al. (2003). "Patients' Responses to Delayed Antibiotic Prescription for Acute Upper Respiratory Tract Infections." *The British Journal of General Practice* 53(496): 845-850.

Elizaga, M. L., R. A. Weinstein, et al. (2002). "Patients in Long-Term Care Facilities: A Reservoir for Vancomycin-Resistant Enterococci." *Clinical Infectious Diseases* 34: 441-446.

Fagon, J. Y., J. Chastre, et al. (2000). "Invasive and Noninvasive Strategies for Management of Suspected Ventilator-Associated Pneumonia. A Randomized Trial." *Annals of Internal Medicine* 132(8): 621-30.

Furuno, J. P., J. C. McGregor, et al. (2006). "Identifying Groups at High Risk for Carriage of Antibiotic-Resistant Bacteria." *Archives of Internal Medicine* 166(5): 580-585.

Fux, C. A., P. Stoodley, et al. (2003). "Bacterial Biofilms: A Diagnostic and Therapeutic Challenge." *Expert Review of Anti-Infective Therapy* 1(4): 667-683.

Hartley, D. M., J. P. Furuno, et al. (2006). "The Role of Institutional Epidemiologic Weight in Guiding Infection Surveillance and Control in Community and Hospital Populations." *Infection Control and Hospital Epidemiology* 27(2): 170-174.

Hayden, M. K., M. J. M. Bonten, et al. (2006). "Reduction in Acquisition of Vancomycin-Resistant Enterococcus After Enforcement of Routine Environmental Cleaning Measures." *Clinical Infectious Diseases* 42(11): 1552-1560.

Henning, K. J., H. Delencastre, et al. (1996). "Vancomycin-Resistant *Enterococcus faecium* on a Pediatric Oncology Ward: Duration of Stool Shedding and Incidence of Clinical Infection." *The Pediatric Infectious Disease Journal* 15: 845-847.

Herold, B. C., L. C. Immergluck, et al. (1998). "Community-Acquired Methicillin-Resistant *Staphylococcus aureus* in Children with No Identified Predisposing Risk." *JAMA* 279(8): 593-598.

HICPAC. (1995). "Recommendations for Preventing the Spread of Vancomycin Resistance. Recommendations of the Hospital Infection Control Practices Advisory Committee (HICPAC)." *MMWR. Recommendations and Reports* 44(RR-12): 13-Jan. Hospital Infection Control Practices Advisory Committee.

Jack, R. W., J. R. Tagg, et al. (1995). "Bacteriocins of Gram-Positive Bacteria." *Microbiological Reviews* 59(2): 171-200.

Kluytmans, J., A. v. Belkam, et al. (1997). "Nasal Carriage of *Staphylococcus aureus*: Epidemiology, Underlying Mechanisms, and Associated Risks." *Clinical Microbiology Reviews* 10: 505-520.

Kluytmans-Vandenbergh, M. F. Q. and J. A. J. W. Kluytmans. (2006). "Community-Acquired Methicillin-Resistant *Staphylococcus aureus*: Current Perspectives." *Clinical Microbiology and Infection* 12 Suppl 1: 15-Sep.

Krause, R. M. (2002). "A Half-Century of Streptococcal Research: Then & Now." *The Indian Journal of Medical Research* 115: 215-241.

Kummerer, K. (2004). "Resistance in the Environment." *The Journal of Antimicrobial Chemotherapy* 54(2): 311-20.

Lange, C. G., A. B. Morrissey, et al. (2000). "Point-Prevalence of Contamination of Health care Workers' Stethoscopes with Vancomycin-Resistant Enterococci at Two Teaching Hospitals in Cleveland, Ohio." *Infection Control and Hospital Epidemiology* 21: 756.

Lessing, M. P., J. Z. Jordens, et al. (1996). "When Should Health care Workers Be Screened for Methicillin-Resistant *Staphylococcus aureus*?" *The Journal of Hospital Infection* 34: 205-210.

Levin, B. R. (2001). "Minimizing Potential Resistance: A Population Dynamics View." *Clinical Infectious Diseases* 33(Suppl 3): S161-S169.

———. (2004). "Microbiology. Noninherited Resistance to Antibiotics." *Science* 305(5690): 1578-1579.

Levin, B. R. and R. Antia. (2001). "Why We Don't Get Sick: The Within-Host Population Dynamics of Bacterial Infections." *Science* 292(5519): 1112-1115.

Levin, B. R., V. E. Perrot, et al. (2000). "Compensatory Mutations, Antibiotic Resistance and the Population Genetics of Adaptive Evolution in Bacteria." *Genetics* 154: 985-997.

Lipsitch, M. (2001). "Measuring and Interpreting Associations Between Antibiotic Use and Penicillin Resistance in *Streptococcus pneumoniae*." *Clinical Infectious Diseases* 32: 1044-1054.

———. (2001). "The Rise and Fall of Antimicrobial Resistance." *Trends in Microbiology* 9: 438-444.

Lipsitch, M., C. T. Bergstrom, et al. (2000). "The Epidemiology of Antibiotic Resistance in Hospitals: Paradoxes and Prescriptions." *Proceedings of the National Academy of Sciences of the United States of America* 97: 1938-1943.

Lipsitch, M. and M. H. Samore. (2002). "Antimicrobial Use and Antimicrobial Resistance: A Population Perspective." *Emerging Infectious Diseases* 8: 347-354.

Lund, B., I. Adamsson, et al. (2002). "Gastrointestinal Transit Survival of an *Enterococcus faecium* Probiotic Strain Administered With or Without Vancomycin." *International Journal of Food Microbiology* 77(2-Jan): 109-115.

Lund, B., C. Agvald-Ohman, et al. (2002). "Frequent Transmission of Enterococcal Strains Between Mechanically Ventilated Patients Treated at an Intensive Care Unit." *Journal of Clinical Microbiology* 40(6): 2084-2088.

Lund, B., C. Edlund, et al. (2000). "Impact on Human Intestinal Microflora of an *Enterococcus faecium* Probiotic and Vancomycin." *Scandinavian Journal of Infectious Diseases* 32(6): 627-632.

Masterton, R. G. (2005). "Antibiotic Cycling: More Than It Might Seem?" *The Journal of Antimicrobial Chemotherapy* 55(1): 5-Jan.

McGowan, J. E., Jr. (1983). "Antimicrobial Resistance in Hospital Organisms and Its Relation to Antibiotic Use." *Reviews of Infectious Diseases* 5(6): 1033-48.

Monnet, D. L. and J. M. Lopez-Lozano. (2005). "Relationship Between Antibiotic Consumption and Resistance in European Hospitals." *Medecine et Maladies Infectieuses* 35 Suppl 2: S127-8.

Nicolle, L. E. (2001). "Preventing Infections in Non-Hospital Settings: Long-Term Care." *Emerging Infectious Diseases* 7(2): 205-207.

O'Brien, T. F. (2002). "Emergence, Spread, and Environmental Effect of Antimicrobial Resistance: How Use of an Antimicrobial Anywhere Can Increase Resistance to Any Antimicrobial Anywhere Else." *Clinical Infectious Diseases.* 34(Suppl 3): S78-S84.

Okeke, I. N. and R. Edelman. (2001). "Dissemination of Antibiotic-Resistant Bacteria Across Geographic Borders." *Clinical Infectious Diseases.* 33: 364-9.

Ostrowsky, B. E., W. E. Trick, et al. (2001). "Control of Vancomycin-Resistant Enterococcus in Health Care Facilities in a Region." *The New England Journal of Medicine* 344: 1427-33.

Paterson, D. L. and L. B. Rice. (2003). "Empirical Antibiotic Choice for the Seriously Ill Patient: Are Minimization of Selection of Resistant Organisms and Maximization of Individual Outcome Mutually Exclusive?" *Clinical Infectious Diseases* 36(8): 1006-1012.

Pelupessy, I., M. J. Bonten, et al. (2002). "How to Assess the Relative Importance of Different Colonization Routes of Pathogens Within Hospital Settings." *Proceedings of the National Academy of Sciences of the United States of America* 99: 5601-5605.

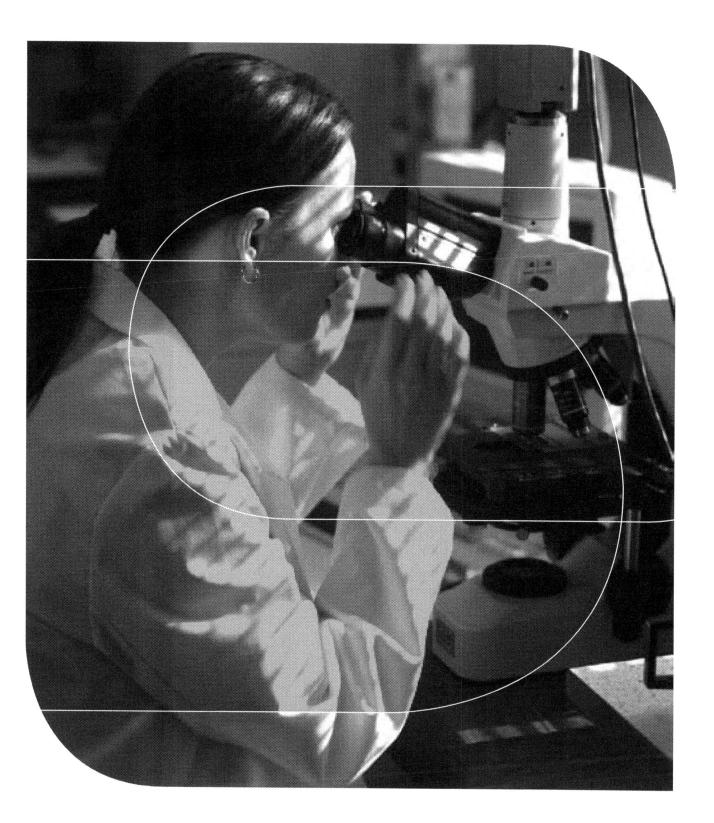

Perencevich, E. N., D. N. Fisman, et al. (2004). "Projected Benefits of Active Surveillance for Vancomycin-Resistant Enterococci in Intensive Care Units." *Clinical Infectious Diseases* 38(8): 1108-15.

Perl, T. M., J. J. Cullen, et al. (2002). "Intranasal Mupirocin to Prevent Postoperative *Staphylococcus aureus* Infections." *The New England Journal of Medicine* 346: 1871-1877.

Phillips, I., M. Casewell, et al. (2004). "Does the Use of Antibiotics in Food Animals Pose a Risk to Human Health? A Critical Review of Published Data." *The Journal of Antimicrobial Chemotherapy* 53: 28-52.

Rice, L. B. (2001). "Emergence of Vancomycin-Resistant Enterococci." *Emerging Infectious Diseases* 7: 183-187.

Riley, M. A. and J. E. Wertz. (2002). "Bacteriocins: Evolution, Ecology, and Application." *Annual Review of Microbiology* 56: 117-137.

Rotun, S. S., V. McMath, et al. (1999). "*Staphylococcus aureus* with Reduced Susceptibility to Vancomycin Isolated From a Patient with Fatal Bacteremia." *Emerging Infectious Diseases* 5(1): 147-149.

Rubin, R. J., C. A. Harrington, et al. (1999). "The Economic Impact of *Staphylococcus aureus* in New York City Hospitals." *Emerging Infectious Diseases* 5(1): 9-17.

Saravolatz, L. D., N. Markowitz, et al. (1982). "Methicillin-Resistant *Staphylococcus aureus.* Epidemiologic Observations During a Community-Acquired Outbreak." *Annals of Internal Medicine* 96(1): 16-Nov.

Saravolatz, L. D., D. J. Pohlod, et al. (1982). "Community-Acquired Methicillin-Resistant *Staphylococcus aureus* Infections: A New Source for Nosocomial Outbreaks." *Annals of Internal Medicine* 97(3): 325-329.

Schrag, S.J., C. Pena, et al. (2001). "Effect of Short-Course, High-Dose Amoxicillin Therapy on Resistant Pneumococcal Carriage: A Randomized Trial." *JAMA* 286(1): 49-56.

Smith, D. L., J. Dushoff, et al. (2004). "Persistent Colonization and the Spread of Antibiotic Resistance in Nosocomial Pathogens: Resistance Is a Regional Problem." *Proceedings of the National Academy of Sciences of the United States of America* 101: 3709-3714.

Smith, D. L., J. Dushoff, et al. (2005). "Agricultural Antibiotics and Human Health." *PLoS Medicine* 2(8): e232.

Smith, D. L., A. D. Harris, et al. (2002). "Animal Antibiotic Use Has an Early But Important Impact on the Emergence of Antibiotic Resistance in Human Commensal Bacteria." *Proceedings of the National Academy of Sciences of the United States of America* 99(9): 6434-9.

Smith, D. L., S. A. Levin, et al. (2005). "Strategic Interactions in Multi-Institutional Epidemics of Antibiotic Resistance." *Proceedings of the National Academy of Sciences of the United States of America* 102: 3153-3158.

Sohn, A. H., B. E. Ostrowsky, et al. (2001). "Evaluation of a Successful Vancomycin-Resistant Enterococcus Prevention Intervention in a Community of Health Care Facilities." *American Journal of Infection Control* 29: 53-7.

Trick, W. E., M. J. Kuehnert, et al. (1999). "Regional Dissemination of Vancomycin-Resistant Enterococci Resulting from Interfacility Transfer of Colonized Patients." *The Journal of Infectious Diseases* 180: 391-396.

Trick, W. E., R. A. Weinstein, et al. (2001). "Colonization of Skilled-Care Facility Residents with Antimicrobial-Resistant Pathogens." *Journal of the American Geriatrics Society* 49: 270-276.

Verhoef, J., D. Beaujean, et al. (1999). "A Dutch Approach to Methicillin-Resistant *Staphylococcus aureus.*" *European Journal of Clinical Microbiology & Infectious Diseases* 18: 461-466.

Vriens, M., H. Blok, et al. (2002). "Costs Associated With a Strict Policy to Eradicate Methicillin-Resistant *Staphylococcus aureus* in a Dutch University Medical Center: A 10-year Survey." *European Journal of Clinical Microbiology & Infectious Diseases* 21: 782-786.

Weinstein, R. A. (2001). "Controlling Antimicrobial Resistance in Hospitals: Infection Control and Use of Antibiotics." *Emerging Infectious Diseases* 7: 188-192.

Witte, W. (1998). "Medical Consequences of Antibiotic Use in Agriculture." *Science* 279: 996-997.`

Wiuff, C., R. M. Zappala, et al. (2005). "Phenotypic Tolerance: Antibiotic Enrichment of Noninherited Resistance in Bacterial Populations." *Antimicrobial Agents and Chemotherapy* 49(4): 1483-1494.

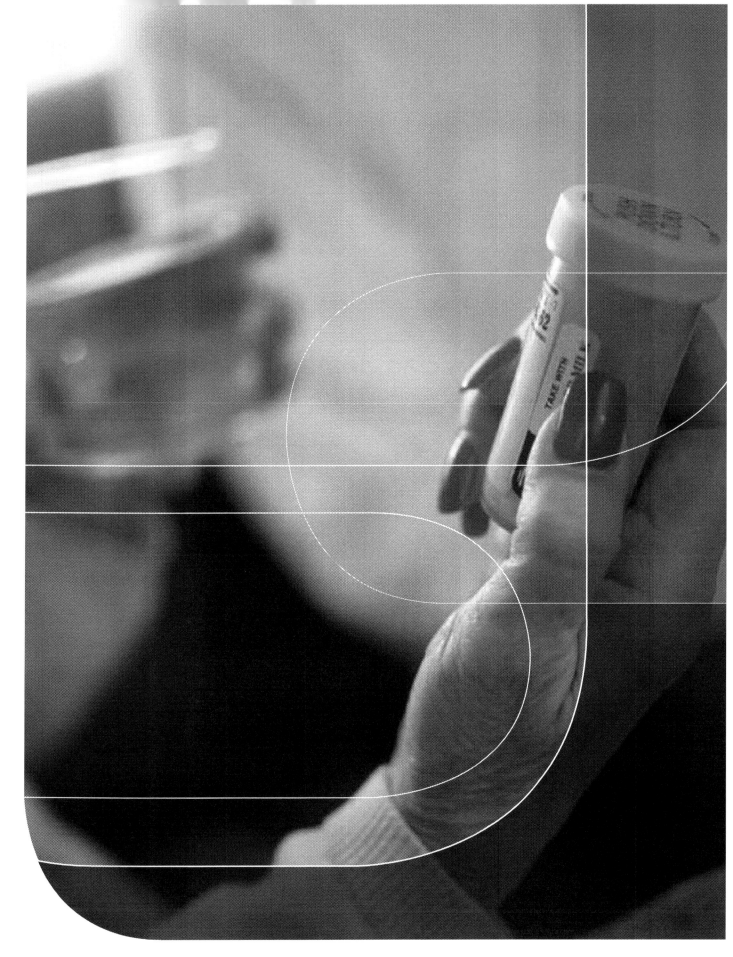

# Patient and physician **demand for antibiotics**

*David Howard*

Interest in understanding patient and physician demand for antibiotics is rooted in the perception that antibiotics are overused, especially in outpatient settings. In the medical literature, "overuse," or "inappropriate use," refers to situations where patients receive antibiotics for conditions that are mostly due to viral pathogens (which are unresponsive to antibiotic treatment) or tend to clear up quickly even if left untreated. In both cases, patients' benefit from antibiotic treatment compared with watchful waiting is minimal or nonexistent. Overuse also occurs if a patient unnecessarily receives a broad-spectrum antibiotic—one that is active against multiple pathogens and typically more effective in treating resistant strains than older, narrow-spectrum drugs (e.g., amoxicillin).

In the economics literature, "overuse" is defined in terms of benefits and costs. The benefit of antibiotic consumption to patients is faster resolution of symptoms and cure. The benefit to society, which is often downplayed in the medical literature on resistance, is reduced transmission of infectious diseases. The cost of consumption, aside from the price of the drug itself, is borne by future generations, who because of resistance will have fewer options for treating infectious diseases. When costs to society exceed benefits to society, an antibiotic is overused. The economic standard for overuse will tend to be more restrictive (i.e., less likely to categorize consumption as inappropriate use) when the costs of antibiotic consumption are large or when consumption reduces transmission. Unfortunately, the empirical relationships between antibiotic use and the benefits and costs to society are not well understood.

## Patient demand

The benefit to patients of using antibiotics includes a faster recovery time and possibly avoidance of severe complications and even death. Costs include the financial cost of the prescription, the risk of allergic reaction, and the development of primary resistance (patients who take antibiotics frequently require more powerful drugs, possibly raising future costs). The presumption in the medical literature is that patients are not well informed about costs and benefits. Most do not understand the difference between viral and bacterial infections (Vanden Eng, Marcus et al. 2003); education-based patient interventions have reduced antibiotic consumption, indicating that lack of knowledge contributes to overuse.

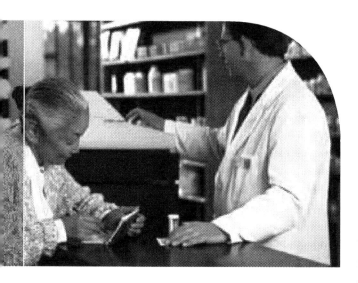

:: PRICES

The standard economic prescription for addressing negative consumption externalities (in this case, antibiotic resistance) is to make the consumer bear the costs of the externality by using a tax (or quotas or permits) to reduce consumption. However, given the availability and wide use of health insurance, it is unclear whether an "antibiotic tax" would have

the desired effect. In most cases, consumers pay only a fixed cost per prescription (usually between $10 and $20), and so the health plan would be directly responsible for paying the tax. The impact of the tax would depend on health plans' responses. If plans pass along some of the tax to consumers in the form of higher copayments, or if plans take additional steps to discourage physicians from prescribing antibiotics, then a tax will reduce consumption. In general, though, the case for using a tax to reduce antibiotic consumption is not as clear-cut as it is in settings where consumer and payer are one and the same.

In place of a tax, government might consider encouraging health plans to increase patients' copayments for antibiotics (Laxminarayan 2003). In recent years there has been a renewed interest in using cost sharing, in the form of "tiered formularies," to influence prescribing behavior and drug consumption. Antibiotics have not been a focus of these efforts, however. Instead, insurers have targeted medications consumed on an ongoing basis, like antihypertensives, and tried to steer patients from brand-name to generic versions. Studies of tiered copayments find that they affect overall consumption and drug choice (Leibowitz, Manning et al. 1985; Hillman, Pauly et al. 1999; Tamblyn, Laprise et al. 2001). Huskamp, Epstein et al. (2003) found that spending and use of certain classes of drugs changed far more when an employer switched from a one-tier to a three-tier formulary with across-the-board increases in copayments than under a more moderate switch, from a two-tier to a three-tier plan with no increase in payments in the first or second tier. Huskamp, Frank et al. (2005) analyzed the change in use of common medications when a health plan changed from a two-tier to a three-tier formulary and found that overall use did not change but that patients were more likely to purchase drugs from the less expensive tier.

The only published study to have evaluated the impact of cost sharing on antibiotic use is the RAND Health Insurance

Experiment, a randomized controlled trial of cost sharing in health care conducted between 1974 and 1982 (Foxman, Valdez et al. 1987). Consumers in the free care plan, where all medical care expenses were covered by insurance, used 85 percent more antibiotics than consumers in plans that required consumers to pay a portion of their medical care bills. Because cost-sharing requirements were applied to all types of services, it was difficult to isolate the impact of cost sharing for antibiotics from the impact of cost sharing for complementary services like physician office visits.

Cost sharing did not appear to differentially reduce antibiotic prescriptions for conditions that were primarily viral, indicating that cost sharing reduced both "appropriate" and "inappropriate" consumption. This finding suggests that cost sharing is a fairly blunt tool for reducing overuse. In theory, health plans could vary cost-sharing amounts based on patients' diagnoses and the appropriateness of the prescription, but this would probably be very difficult to implement in practice.

Given current price levels for commonly used antibiotics, the potential for increased copayments for antibiotics to reduce demand is limited. Many commonly prescribed antibiotics, such as amoxicillin, cost less than $20 per course, and so at current copayment levels consumers are already paying a large share of the price, if not the entire amount, out of pocket. For some off-patent antibiotics, patients' copayments may actually exceed the wholesale price of the drug.

Cost sharing may be an effective tool to induce consumers to switch from newer, more expensive antibiotics to older drugs (if that were a goal), but evidence on the magnitude of the effect is lacking. Clinical guidelines frequently recommend that broad-spectrum drugs be held in reserve, though this policy diminishes incentives for research and development of new antibiotics and may even contribute to the development of antibiotic resistance by loading selection pressure on a handful of older drugs (see Chapter 7 for a detailed discussion).

Health plans that require higher cost sharing for both drugs and office visits, such as health care savings accounts, may be more successful in reducing demand for antibiotics. Such plans, which are marketed as "consumer driven," have gained in popularity in recent years. The RAND study concluded that "the effect of cost sharing on antibiotic use comes principally through a reduction in visits rather than as a result of reduced antibiotic prescribing given a visit" (Foxman, Valdez et al. 1987).

## :: DISPENSING RESTRICTIONS

Cost sharing is not the only way to raise the "price" of antibiotics to consumers. Policies that make it more difficult for patients to obtain antibiotics—for example, by prohibiting physicians from directly dispensing antibiotics—may reduce consumption even among patients who receive prescriptions. A recent study found that antibiotic prescribing for viral illness in Korea declined by eight percentage points after a 2000 law was passed prohibiting physician dispensing (Park, Soumerai et al. 2005). Physician dispensing of antibiotics is not as widespread in the United States as it is in Asia, and so banning U.S. physician dispensing may have only a small impact. Another policy is to give physicians the option of issuing antibiotic prescriptions with waiting periods: basically, the prescription would entitle patients to receive antibiotics a certain number of days or hours following the physician office visit. This approach permits physicians to acknowledge patients' symptoms and distress via the prescription but imposes an additional barrier between the receipt of the prescription and the dispensing of the antibiotic. It is consistent with sound clinical practice—patients whose symptoms persist will fill the prescription, while patients whose symptoms resolve probably did not need the antibiotic in the first place—and does not impose additional costs on the health care system, since patients are not required to return for a follow-up visit once the waiting period is over.

## :: PROMOTING SUBSTITUTES

Promotion of substitutes to antibiotics is another strategy for reducing use, one that may be more politically palatable than policies that make it more difficult or costly for patients to obtain antibiotics. The economic rationale for promoting substitutes is obvious, but it is also worth noting that this approach to reducing antibiotic demand is consistent with anthropological theories of overprescribing. These emphasize the role of prescriptions in signaling the end to a physician encounter. Once patients have gone to the trouble of visiting a physician or emergency room, they may feel entitled to an antibiotic prescription (Macfarlane, Holmes et al. 1997; Kumar, Little et al. 2003). Use of substitutes affords physicians the opportunity to "do something" about patients' complaints and acknowledge their validity without having to prescribe an antibiotic that they know will be ineffective.

Government and health plans could increase the use of substitutes by decreasing their price to consumers. For example, a health plan could dispense free or heavily discounted "cold kits" to physicians, who can give them to patients with respiratory symptoms as a substitute for an antibiotic prescription. The kits might contain decongestants, nasal sprays, and cough drops. At least one health plan attempted this strategy but found it costly, time-consuming, and of limited effectiveness in reducing antibiotic use. Many of the kits were taken by persons outside the target group (e.g., receptionists). Currently, Pfizer Consumer Health Care, manufacturer of Sudafed, distributes cold kits to physicians over the Internet (see http://www.aware.md/ed_materials/cold_kits.asp).

Policies that increase consumers' access to substitutes may help patients avoid a visit to the doctor's office. For example, the Food and Drug Administration could shift some products from prescription to over-the-counter status, making it possible for consumers to obtain antibiotic substitutes without a physician visit.

> Policies that increase consumers' access to substitutes may help patients avoid a visit to the doctor's office.

States may also want to reconsider policy changes to limit access to over-the-counter decongestants that contain pseudoephedrine, a crucial ingredient in "crystal meth." In some cases pharmacies are voluntarily removing or are required by state law to remove decongestants with pseudoephedrine from shelves to behind the pharmacy counter. A pending federal law would require purchasers to sign a log book. Though requiring patients to ask pharmacists for decongestants does not seem to present a significant barrier to legitimate users, many manufacturers are nevertheless reformulating products, substituting phenylephrine for pseudoephedrine. Phenylephrine must be taken more frequently than pseudoephedrine and it may not be as effective (Johannes 2005).

The lack of effectiveness of alternatives to antibiotics is a major obstacle to promoting substitutes. Evidence that decongestants and other over-the-counter remedies relieve cold symptoms is limited. Decongestants and antihistamines have been shown to be ineffective in relieving symptoms from acute otitis media in children (Flynn, Griffin et al. 2004). A review of more than 35 published studies found no evidence to support the use of antihistamines alone as a remedy for the common cold, and although in combination with decongestants they displayed a beneficial effect in a majority of the studies, it was unclear whether the results were clinically significant (Sutter, Lemiengre et al. 2003).

Arroll (2005) reviewed several studies on nonantibiotic cold remedies—antihistamines, decongestants, *Echinacea,* humidification, and others—and found that only one, rest, was at all useful; he also found that antibiotics have no effect on the severity of the common cold. Paul, Yoder et al. (2004) also found little evidence that over-the-counter cough medicine improves symptoms or sleep quality among children with coughs.

Symptoms of respiratory infections may also be alleviated with nonpharmacological treatments, such as nasal irrigation. Although clinical trials have indicated that irrigation may be successful in treating chronic sinusitis (Tomooka, Murphy et al. 2000; Rabago, Zgierska et al. 2002), its efficacy in treating the common cold or acute bacterial rhinosinusitis is unclear (Adam, Stiffman et al. 1998; Rabago, Barrett et al. 2005).

## :: PATIENT EDUCATION

Previous efforts to reduce patient demand have tended to emphasize the role of information and education. If patients overestimate the benefit of antibiotics, then providing information about the effectiveness of antibiotics for specific conditions and symptoms may reduce demand. Because patient educational interventions are usually coupled with interventions directed at physicians, it is difficult to isolate the impact of patient education. A recent review of the literature found that studies of combined patient and physician interventions did not report larger effect sizes than studies of physician interventions alone (Ranji, Steinman et al. 2006). (We review this literature in more depth in the next section.)

A handful of studies have examined the impact of patient education alone. Macfarlane, Holmes et al. (2002) randomized patients with acute bronchitis to receive usual care or literature explaining the possible negative consequences of taking antibiotics and an oral message that in most cases antibiotics would do little good. This intervention reduced antibiotic use

by 25 percent. Gonzales, Steiner et al. (1999) report that the addition of a patient education component to an ongoing physician education campaign was associated with a slight decline in prescribing rates in pediatric practices but a large reduction in prescribing rates for adult patients. Taylor, Kwan-Gett et al. (2003) found that educational materials distributed to parents on the judicious use of antibiotics had no effect on prescribing rates, though these researchers did not measure actual prescriptions filled or consumption.

## :: PREVENTION AND VACCINATION

In inpatient settings, strategies to address the spread of resistance focus primarily on reducing the incidence and transmission of disease through hygiene and patient isolation. Prevention has been less of a focus in the community—there are so many more conduits for transmission—but it is the most direct method for reducing antibiotic demand, and unlike policies to reduce use of antibiotics, it does not pose the political and ethical challenges of withholding potentially effective medical care from sick patients. Schools and day-care clinics often require that sick children be kept home, and some employers also require that sick persons stay home. The

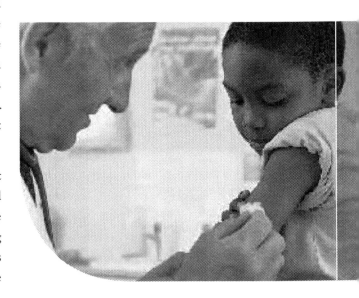

effect on antibiotic use is unknown. On the one hand, it may reduce transmission. On the other, it may increase demand for antibiotics among people eager to return to work or see their children return to school.

Vaccination with pneumococcal conjugate vaccine and influenza vaccine has also been promoted as a policy to reduce disease incidence, antibiotic demand, and resistance. Predicting the impact of long-term mass vaccination is difficult, but findings from clinical trials (Jacobs 2002) and epidemiological surveillance studies (Whitney, Farley et al. 2003) suggest that pneumococcal vaccination is effective in reducing incidence of pneumococcal disease and incidence of infection with resistant strains (Klugman 2004; Talbot, Poehling et al. 2004; Poehling, Talbot et al. 2006); the vaccine is differentially active against drug-resistant serotypes. In addition, there appears to be a spillover benefit from vaccination to nonvaccinated hosts (Whitney, Farley et al. 2003).

Vaccination creates opportunities for transmission of and infection with nonpneumococcal pathogens and nonvaccine serotypes of *Streptococcus pneumoniae* (Kyaw, Lynfield et al. 2006). Three trials of pneumococcal vaccination found that rates of acute otitis media did not differ or were only slightly lower in the treatment group compared with controls (Jacobs 2002), but it is conceivable that widespread vaccination could lower incidence rates over a longer timeframe. Many studies of the impact of influenza vaccination in children have found that vaccination reduces the risk of otitis media (see, e.g., Belshe, Mendelman et al. 1998), but not all studies have reached this conclusion (Hoberman, Greenberg et al. 2003).

If vaccination is shown to be an effective strategy for reducing the incidence of infection (and, consequently, use of antibiotics), then it will be important to consider new policies for increasing vaccination uptake. The government can require that all school-age children receive pneumococcal vaccinations. In the absence of a mandate, the government may need to offer subsidies or impose coverage mandates on insurers to significantly increase uptake. Currently, pneumococcal vaccination is relatively expensive compared with other common vaccines, and not all health plans cover pneumococcal vaccination.

■ _____

## Physician demand

In the short term, physicians' incentives to prescribe antibiotics will depend on the reimbursement system and the internal reward structure of the physician group. Most primary-care physicians practice in groups, and so the financial incentives for the group as a whole may differ substantially from those for individual physicians, though one would expect group managers to align group and individual incentives as closely as possible.

Most groups are compensated using either fee-for-service reimbursement or capitation. Under fee-for-service reimbursement, groups are paid a per-visit fee. Under capitation, groups are paid a per-member per-month fee. In general, fee-for-service reimbursement is associated with stronger incentives to treat patients aggressively, while capitation presents incentives to treat patients conservatively, though the opposite may be true in situations where aggressive treatment means referring patients to specialists not covered under the capitation contract.

The impact of these alternative reimbursement arrangements on physicians to prescribe antibiotics depends on whether antibiotics are a substitute for, or complement to, follow-up visits. Most likely, antibiotics and follow-up visits are substitutes; physicians instruct patients who receive antibiotics to take the full course of the drug before making another visit. Patients who do not receive antibiotics may be advised to return for a follow-up visit in a few days if symptoms persist. When antibiotics and follow-up visits are substitutes, fee-for-service reimbursement will be associated with lower rates

> # Studies have found that physicians with greater workloads are more likely to prescribe antibiotics.

of antibiotic prescribing, and capitation with higher rates. Evidence on the degree to which antibiotics and follow-up visits are substitutes or complements is limited. One study found that a large decrease in antibiotic prescribing rates following a physician and patient educational intervention was not associated with an increase in return visits (Gonzales, Steiner et al. 1999), but another study, in which patients were randomized to treatment (immediate antibiotics, delayed antibiotics, no antibiotics), found that 19 percent of patients in the no-antibiotic group returned for a follow-up visit, compared with 11 percent of patients in the immediate-antibiotic group (Little, Rumsby et al. 2005).

Within physician groups, a portion of physicians' pay may be tied to "productivity," which is often measured by the number of patients seen. The medical and sociological literature on antibiotic prescribing and inappropriate prescribing in general emphasizes that physicians can use prescriptions as a tool for reducing the length of office visits. The prescription signals to the patient that the visit is concluded, and it indicates that the physician understands and recognizes the legitimacy of the patient's complaints (Steinke, MacDonald et al. 1999). If a practice operates at full capacity, a physician who sees more patients during the day may earn a productivity-based bonus. If a practice operates at less than full capacity, physicians who finish their appointments ahead of schedule can spend the rest of their workday on administrative tasks or go home early. Studies have found that physicians with greater workloads are more likely to prescribe antibiotics (Gonzales, Steiner et al. 1997; Hutchinson and Foley 1997; Arnold, Allen et al. 1999).

Explaining to patients why they do not need antibiotics can take as long as 10 to 15 minutes—valuable time to a busy physician.

Although reimbursement and bonus incentives have been found to play an important role in influencing practice patterns in a variety of settings, the medical literature on overprescribing tends to downplay short-term financial considerations. Instead, survey and focus group results emphasize the role of patient demand (Schwartz, Soumerai et al. 1989; Barden, Dowell et al. 1998; APUA 1999; Bauchner, Pelton et al. 1999; Metlay, Shea et al. 2002). Physicians fear that if they do not meet patients' expectations, they will lose patients to other practices. Survey results must be interpreted cautiously. Responses reflect survey structure, and so a survey that asks physicians about the role of patient demand but not reimbursement may mischaracterize the nonclinical factors responsible for overprescribing. The survey that included the most comprehensive list of factors influencing prescribing (APUA 1999) found that 59 percent of respondents cited patient demand, but only 26 percent cited time pressure and 20 percent cited the potential for a return visit (respondents were allowed multiple responses). Also, such studies measure physicians' perceptions of patient behavior, not actual behavior. We are not aware of any studies showing that patients switch physicians if they are refused antibiotics. A study that analyzed actual patient-physician interactions found that explicit demands for antibiotics by patients are rare (Stivers 2002a). Other studies have found that physicians perceive patient demand for antibiotics when there is none (Mangione-Smith, McGlynn et al. 1999) and that patient demand is more often implicit (e.g., suggesting a diagnosis) than explicit (Stivers 2002b). Nevertheless, "patient demand" is usually cited by physicians as the most important factor contributing to overuse, and there are anecdotal reports of patients' demanding specific, broad-spectrum antibiotics.

The use of "patient satisfaction" tools may reinforce the

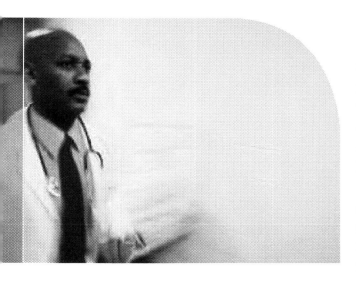

incentive to please patients by prescribing antibiotics. Some health plans use patient satisfaction measures in contracting decisions or to determine bonus payments. Other plans release satisfaction scores directly to patients, who may use the information when selecting physicians. Little, Rumsby et al. (2005) found that when patients with lower respiratory tract infections were randomized to receive an immediate antibiotic, a delayed antibiotic, or no antibiotic, the proportion of patients who were very satisfied was 14 percent higher in the immediate-antibiotic group than in the no-antibiotic group. A study by Christakis, Wright et al. (2005) reported that parents were more satisfied when their children received antibiotics for cough and cold symptoms, and a survey of parents found that 40 percent would be somewhat or extremely dissatisfied if watchful waiting was recommended (Finkelstein, Stille et al. 2005). Other work suggests that the time spent with the physician (Ranji, Steinman et al. 2006) or physician-patient communication (Mangione-Smith, McGlynn et al. 1999), rather than receipt of an antibiotic, is a more important determinant of patient satisfaction. Gonzales, Steiner et al. (2001) found that a combined patient and physician education effort lowered antibiotic consumption but did not adversely affect patients' satisfaction with care.

Fear of malpractice lawsuits is sometimes cited as a factor contributing to overprescribing. A child who suffers from meningitis that could have been averted with an antibiotic prescription would make a sympathetic victim. However, there are no documented cases in the medical literature of a physician being sued for failing to prescribe an antibiotic, and a board member of a malpractice insurer reported that he was unaware of such cases (Kenneth E. Thorpe, personal communication, May 3, 2006). In surveys, physicians do not rate liability concerns highly compared with other nonclinical factors driving inappropriate antibiotic use APUA 1999; Bauchner, Pelton et al. 1999). The prospect of lawsuits is, however, an emerging issue in inpatient settings (see Chapter 4), where lax hand washing and poor hygiene contribute to the spread of both resistant and sensitive bacteria.

## :: PAY FOR PERFORMANCE

Over the past several years, many health plans have started to use bonuses tied to quality measures, or "pay for performance" programs, to influence physician behavior. Quality measures are typically based on patient satisfaction surveys, measures of physicians' adherence to medical practice guidelines, or even patients' outcomes. Antibiotic prescribing is not a focus of these efforts, which instead emphasize cancer screening and quality and process measures for chronic conditions like diabetes. Although there is a great deal of enthusiasm among payers, employers, and policymakers for pay-for-performance programs, it can be surprisingly difficult to design effective incentive schemes. Rosenthal, Frank et al. (2005) studied a pay-for-performance program in a California health plan that rewarded physician groups based on the level of cervical cancer screening, breast cancer screening, and hemoglobin A1c testing. They found that the program basically rewarded physician groups whose levels were high to begin with, and improvements in quality were apparent for only one of three measures. Pay for performance can also lead physicians to avoid high-risk or noncompliant patients or overuse certain technologies. For example, programs that measure quality based on cancer screening rates may lead physicians to recommend screening for older, sicker persons who are unlikely to benefit from early detection (Walter, Davidowitz et al. 2004).

Quality bonuses could potentially be used to influence antibiotic prescribing rates. It would be difficult, however, to differentiate between appropriate and inappropriate prescribing in such a way as to discourage miscoding and misclassification. Diagnoses for acute respiratory conditions are somewhat interchangeable, so it is simple for physicians to substitute an "appropriate" ICD-9 code for an "inappropriate" code when bonus funds are at stake. In some cases the appropriateness of prescribing an antibiotic depends on symptom duration, which is not recorded in insurers' administrative claims files.

Even if patients' complaints were documented accurately in administrative data, it is unclear how to link bonuses to physician behavior. Should bonuses be tied to absolute prescribing levels or changes in prescribing patterns? Should bonuses be tied to the number of prescriptions or prescribing rates (i.e., the number of prescriptions divided by the number of patients seeking treatment for colds, ear infections, etc.)? Each option presents problems. For example, tying payments to prescribing rates may lead physicians to encourage patients with minor symptoms to seek care, thereby inflating the denominator of the prescribing rate ratio.

## :: ELECTRONIC MEDICAL RECORDS

Continued use of an antibiotic or use of antibiotics from a given class increases the risk that patients will develop primary resistance. Prescribing guidelines, such as the Infectious Diseases Society of America's (IOSA) guideline for pneumonia (Bartlett, Breiman et al. 1998), recommend that physicians select an antibiotic from a different class for patients who recently received antibiotics. For example,

if a patient received a macrolide previously, the physician should prescribe a penicillin or cephalosporin for the next prescription. Analysis of prescribing patterns indicates that the recommendation to rotate or switch antibiotics is often not followed in practice (Wu, Howard et al. 2006). One of the difficulties in adhering to the guideline is that physicians may be unaware of the types of antibiotics that patients have been prescribed previously. Electronic medical records, which follow patients across settings, may help improve prescribing patterns by allowing physicians to access past medications. Electronic records could be programmed with electronic flags to alert physicians when they do not prescribe guideline-recommended therapy. Also, patients who use a large number of antibiotics over a certain period could be targeted for special educational interventions or even subjected to higher cost-sharing amounts.

From a societal standpoint, electronic records would be useful for surveillance and for implementing mixed prescribing strategies (Laxminarayan and Weitzman 2002), where many antibiotics are used simultaneously to avoid excessive selection pressure on any particular antibiotic or antibiotic class. Although it is not clear how a mixed strategy could be enforced across settings or payers, large clinics or health plans could use electronic record systems to encourage and monitor adherence with mixed prescribing for their patients and enrollees. For example, a clinic could add a prompt to electronic medical records that randomly assigns penicillin-based antibiotics for some patients and macrolides for others with a given condition, taking into account patients' allergies and recent antibiotic usage.

## :: MANAGING DRUG COMPANY–PHYSICIAN INTERACTIONS

Pharmaceutical company marketing, which encompasses print advertising and physician detailing, has both brand-expanding and business-stealing effects. For antibiotics, which are a mature product, we can assume that marketing has been primarily a business-stealing effect. There is little

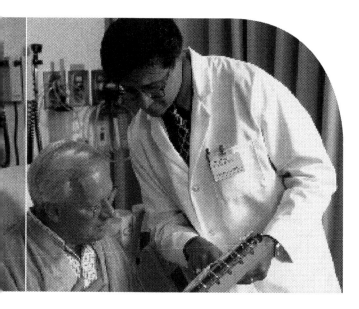

information on the magnitude of companies' marketing efforts on behalf of antibiotics. A casual inspection of pediatric and family medicine journals indicates that antibiotics are advertised and that many of the advertisements are for broad-spectrum drugs. Many advertisements make reference to the drug's activity against resistant strains. Companies also promote antibiotics with physician detailing (i.e., interactions between companies' sales forces and physicians) and by distributing samples.

To the extent that marketing leads to overuse of antibiotics and broad-spectrum drugs in particular, policies to counteract the impact of advertising and detailing may slow the development of resistant strains. "Academic detailing" (or alternatively, "counter detailing") is generally considered the most effective educational method of influencing prescribing patterns (Gross and Pujat 2001; Bloom 2005). In academic detailing, a representative from a neutral organization, such as a professional society, hospital, or public health agency, meets with physicians one-on-one to discuss prescribing practices (Soumerai and Avorn 1990). Typically, the detailer

is a peer or someone knowledgeable in the clinical area being discussed and is trained in effective communication. Academic detailing has been used successfully to reduce overuse of several types of drug classes (Soumerai and Avorn 1990; Bloom 2005), including antibiotics (Gross and Pujat 2001; Solomon, Van Houten et al. 2001).

## :: INTERVENTIONS TO IMPROVE DIAGNOSTIC ACCURACY

Though most physicians recognize that antibiotics are overprescribed in aggregate, it is not easy to determine the appropriateness of antibiotics for individual patients. Few physicians can rule out bacterial infection with certainty based on the often nonspecific complaints of patients suffering from respiratory conditions. There is always a chance that antibiotics will help, and in rare cases failure to prescribe antibiotics may lead to serious complications, like meningitis.

Development of decision rules and diagnostic tests that enable physicians to determine the etiology of infections and symptoms can reduce use of antibiotics and broad-spectrum drugs. Decision rules employ easily observable patient characteristics to predict the response to antibiotic therapy. Though most decision rules have fairly low sensitivity and specificity, they are inexpensive and can be easily incorporated into clinical practice. Diagnostic tests are more accurate but are also more expensive and invasive. Several promising tests are under development (Christ-Crain, Jaccard-Stolz et al. 2004; Esposito, Tremolati et al. 2005), but most currently available tests are too slow or entail too much discomfort to patients to be of much practical use in office settings.

## :: PHYSICIAN EDUCATION AND QUALITY IMPROVEMENT

Most ongoing efforts to reduce antibiotic prescribing use various types of educational interventions and "quality improvement" strategies targeted at physicians and patients. Educational materials typically describe situations where antibiotic prescribing is and is not appropriate and attempt to raise physicians' awareness of the problem of resistance. Strategies to disseminate information include educational mailings to physicians, educational pamphlets for patients, and academic detailing (discussed above).

Since 1995 the Centers for Disease Control and Prevention has funded a national educational campaign to reduce overuse (see http://www.cdc.gov/drugresistance/community/). Originally named the National Campaign for Appropriate Antibiotic Use in the Community and renamed Get Smart, this program focuses on changing prescribing patterns for patients with upper respiratory infections and targets providers, patients, and parents. National trends in prescribing rates and antibiotic use suggest that it and similar efforts to raise awareness about the problem of resistance have been effective. From 1980 to 1992, antibiotic use rates in the population increased (though the increases were not statistically significant at the 5 percent level) (McCaig and Hughes 1995). In more recent years, however, studies have documented substantial declines in antibiotic use (McCaig, Besser et al. 2002; Finkelstein, Stille et al. 2003; Steinman, Gonzales et al. 2003; Stille, Andrade et al. 2004; Roumie, Halasa et al. 2005; Miller and Hudson 2006). For example, McCaig, Besser et al. (2002) report that the number of antibiotics prescribed annually in physicians' offices to children under age 15 declined from 45.5 million in 1989–1990 to 30.3 million in 1999–2000. Prescribing rates declined from 838 per 1,000 children to 503 per 1,000 children. Likewise, Steinman, Gonzales et al. (2003) report that the proportion of outpatient visits where the patient received an antibiotic decreased from 13 percent to 10 percent between 1991–1992 and 1989–1999 for adults and from 33 percent to 22 percent for children. The total number of antibiotic prescriptions decreased from 230 million to 190 million. While antibiotic use has declined, however, the market share of broad-spectrum drugs has been increasing (Steinman, Gonzales et al. 2003; Stille, Andrade et al. 2004).

Howard (2005) argues that concerns about resistance are partly responsible for the shift toward broad-spectrum drugs. Thus, efforts to publicize the impact of overuse on patient outcomes will decrease antibiotic use overall but may have the unintended consequence of increasing consumption of broad-spectrum antibiotics.

Programs to reduce antibiotic use may be effective in reducing rates of resistance among the most common respiratory pathogen, *Streptococcus pneumoniae*. Recent surveillance data indicate that although resistance to fluoroquinolones is becoming more common in *S. pneumoniae*, resistance to other drug classes is decreasing (Doern, Richter et al. 2005). This pattern is consistent with trends in prescribing patterns. A French study reported that region-level interventions to reduce antibiotic use were associated with reductions in the rate of colonization with penicillin-resistant *S. pneumoniae* (Guillemot, Varon et al. 2005).

Controlled studies of educational interventions provide additional evidence on the effectiveness of education and quality improvement. Unlike studies of antibiotic use trends, they control for other factors that may affect antibiotic use over time (e.g., publicity surrounding the "hygiene hypothesis," which posits that lack of early exposure to pathogens leads to immune-related disorders later in life). A

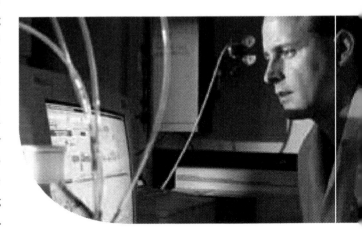

recent summary of these studies concluded that educational interventions, which are often accompanied by feedback, reduced prescribing rates by about 9 percent and increased adherence to guidelines on antibiotic choice by more than 10 percent (Ranji, Steinman et al. 2006). To put these results in perspective, the review noted, "For a 100,000-member health maintenance organization (HMO), these studies suggest that a QI [quality improvement] strategy targeting all ARIs [antibiotic-resistant infections] for patients of all age groups would result in a savings of approximately 3000 to 8000 antibiotic prescriptions per year."

Studies that combined profiling and education did not report better results than studies of education alone. Educational interventions that employed active learning strategies, like academic detailing, led to larger reductions than interventions that relied on passive learning strategies, like mailings—a finding echoed in earlier reviews (Gross and Pujat 2001; Sbarbaro 2001). As mentioned above, studies with a patient education component did not report better results than studies that examined only physician education.

The median duration of studies included in the Ranji, Steinman et al. review (2006) was only six months, raising concerns about the durability of the interventions. At the population level, the reductions in antibiotic use noted earlier have been sustained, suggesting that even if the effect of a single, small-scale intervention is reversible, the cumulative effect of multiple interventions and nationwide education efforts is not. Based on the published literature to date, it is difficult to determine whether interventions to reduce antibiotic use are cost-effective.

Going forward, it is unclear whether additional educational programs can further reduce antibiotic prescribing rates. Gonzales, Corbett et al. (2005) studied the impact of a recent educational initiative in Colorado. They concluded that although the program reduced antibiotic prescribing rates for adult patients, "there appears to be little room for improvement in antibiotic prescription rates for children with pharyngitis." A study of the same intervention, limited to elderly enrollees in a Medicare managed care plan, found that it did not affect prescribing rates in this population. (Gonzales, Sauaia et al. 2004)

## Conclusion and issues for future research

Policies to reduce antibiotic use in outpatient settings can appeal to extrinsic motivations (i.e., self-interest), intrinsic motivations (i.e., wanting to do good for its own sake), or a combination of both. Policies that appeal to extrinsic motivation include cost sharing and pay for performance. Policies that appeal to intrinsic motivations include education and feedback. Historically, policies to reduce antibiotic use and improve health care quality more generally have relied on intrinsic motivation based on the theory that physicians want to do the right thing—they just lack information and the right tools. Along the same lines, poor quality was viewed as a manifestation of poorly designed systems, rather than the fault of specific individuals. In the past few years, attitudes toward quality improvement have shifted somewhat, and appeals to clinicians' and patients' extrinsic motivations are becoming more common. Policies that rely on extrinsic motivation are often powerful, but there is always the risk that appeals to pecuniary motives may crowd out intrinsic motivations. Also, policies that appeal to extrinsic motivations can lead to unintended consequences. For example, as discussed earlier, a policy to tie compensation to prescribing rates could lead physicians to encourage visits by patients with minor symptoms to make the prescribing rate appear to be lower.

Evidence from clinical trials and national trends in prescribing patterns suggests that policies designed to appeal to intrinsic motivations, such as intensive physician and patient education, have led to substantial reductions in antibiotic use. It is unclear whether additional interventions or policy changes are necessary.

The decline in antibiotic use may not be sustainable, or it may be sustainable but further reductions in antibiotic use may be difficult to achieve through educational programs alone.

Price-based interventions, including changes in demand-side cost sharing by patients and the use of bonuses for physicians tied to practice patterns, are an increasingly popular method of lowering costs in primary care. Antibiotic use has not been a focus of these efforts, and aside from the RAND Health Insurance Experiment, their impact on antibiotic use is untested. Research from other clinical areas suggests that price-based interventions have an impact on physician and patient behavior, but incentives are a blunt instrument, and it can be difficult to structure incentives to bring about desired results. With antibiotics, incentive-based programs may fail to differentiate between "appropriate" and "inappropriate" use and can be subject to gaming by physicians. Interventions to make substitutes for antibiotics more readily available, perhaps by giving physicians "cold relief packs" to distribute in their offices, may lower prescribing rates without adversely affecting patient outcomes. The impact of making substitutes to antibiotics more readily available and other nonprice interventions to change the relative cost of antibiotics to patients has not been well studied.

Use of policies to reduce transmission of bacteria and viruses in the community has received little attention in the medical literature, though there is an extensive literature on infection control in inpatient settings. Perhaps clinicians perceive that opportunities for reducing transmission rates are limited, or that it is impossible to marshal public support for meaningful changes unless the disease in question is life threatening. Currently, many day-care centers require parents to keep sick children home. The net impact on antibiotic demand is unknown, since parents may seek antibiotics to speed their children's return (and their own return to work). Vaccination presents an attractive mechanism for reducing antibiotic demand, since in most cases private and public incentives

# Incentive programs may fail to differentiate between "appropriate" use and "inappropriate" use.

for obtaining vaccination are aligned (though not necessarily of the same magnitude). Future work should examine the potential of pneumococcal vaccination for reducing resistance rates directly, via the vaccine's differential activity against resistant serotypes, and indirectly via the impact of the vaccine on antibiotic demand.

An important goal for policy, besides reducing the level of antibiotic use, is improving patterns of use. The medical literature emphasizes the need to hold broad-spectrum antibiotics in reserve, using them only when older drugs have failed, but the emerging economics literature on resistance finds that mixed prescribing strategies are optimal. Designing policies to improve prescribing patterns and implement mixed prescribing strategies is an important goal for future research. Electronic medical records, which allow third parties to monitor prescribing patterns across settings and physicians offices, may be helpful in this regard.

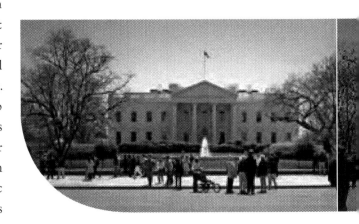

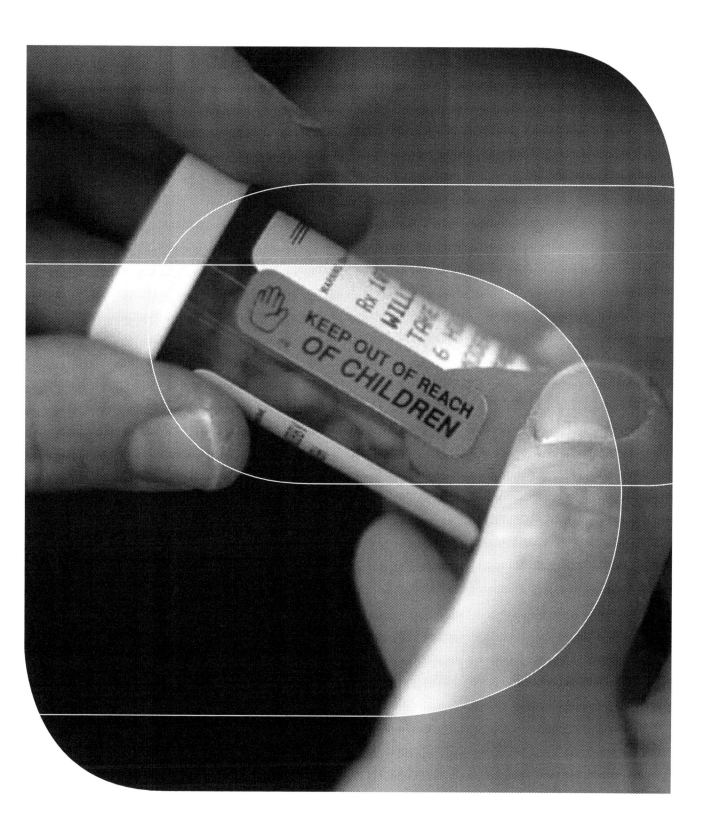

# References

Adam, P., M. Stiffman, et al. (1998). "A Clinical Trial of Hypertonic Saline Nasal Spray in Subjects with the Common Cold or Rhinosinusitis." *Archives of Family Medicine* 7(1): 39-43.

APUA (1999). *Massachusetts Physician Survey. Pilot Survey of Primary Care Physicians in Massachusetts, 1998.* http://www.tufts.edu/med/apua/ Research/physicianSurvey1-01/physicianSurvey.htm (accessed March 9, 2006). Alliance for the Prudent Use of Antibiotics.

Arnold, S. R., U. D. Allen, et al. (1999). "Antibiotic Prescribing by Pediatricians for Respiratory Tract Infection in Children." *Clinical Infectious Diseases* 29(2): 312-17.

Arroll, B. (2005). "Antibiotics for Upper Respiratory Tract Infections: An Overview of Cochrane Reviews." *Respiratory Medicine* 99(3): 255-61.

Barden, L. S., S. F. Dowell, et al. (1998). "Current Attitudes Regarding Use of Antimicrobial Agents: Results from Physician's and Parents' Focus Group Discussions." *Clinical Pediatrics* 37(11): 665-71.

Bartlett, J. G., R. F. Breiman, et al. (1998). "Community-Acquired Pneumonia in Adults: Guidelines for Management." *Clinical Infectious Diseases* 26(4): 811-38.

Bauchner, H., S. I. Pelton, et al. (1999). "Parents, Physicians, and Antibiotic Use." *Pediatrics* 103(2): 395-401.

Belshe, R. B., P. M. Mendelman, et al. (1998). "The Efficacy of Live Attenuated, Cold-Adapted, Trivalent, Intranasal Influenzavirus Vaccine in Children." *The New England Journal of Medicine* 338(20): 1405-12.

Bloom, B. S. (2005). "Effects of Continuing Medical Education on Improving Physician Clinical Care and Patient Health: A Review of Systematic Reviews." *International Journal of Technology Assessment in Health Care* 21(3): 380-5.

Christ-Crain, M., D. Jaccard-Stolz, et al. (2004). "Effect of Procalcitonin-Guided Treatment on Antibiotic Use and Outcome in Lower Respiratory Tract Infections: Cluster-Randomised, Single-Blinded Intervention Trial." *Lancet* 363(9409): 600-7.

Christakis, D. A., J. A. Wright, et al. (2005). "Association Between Parental Satisfaction and Antibiotic Prescription for Children with Cough and Cold Symptoms." *The Pediatric Infectious Disease Journal* 24(9): 774-7.

Doern, G. V., S. S. Richter, et al. (2005). "Antimicrobial Resistance Among *Streptococcus pneumoniae* in the United States: Have We Begun to Turn the Corner on Resistance to Certain Antimicrobial Classes?" *Clinical Infectious Diseases* 41(2):139-48.

Esposito, S., E. Tremolati, et al. (2005). "Evaluation of a Rapid Bedside Test for the Quantitative Determination of C-reactive Protein." *Clinical Chemistry and Laboratory Medicine* 43(4): 438-40.

Finkelstein, J. A., C. Stille, et al. (2003). "Reduction in Antibiotic Use Among US Children, 1996-2000." *Pediatrics* 112(3): 620-627.

Finkelstein, J. A., C. J. Stille, et al. (2005). "Watchful Waiting for Acute Otitis Media: Are Parents and Physicians Ready?" *Pediatrics* 115(6): 1466-73.

Flynn, C. A., G. H. Griffin, et al. (2004). "Decongestants and Antihistamines for Acute Otitis Media in Children." *Cochrane Database of Systematic Reviews* (3): CD001727.

Foxman, B., R. B. Valdez, et al. (1987). "The Effect of Cost Sharing on the Use of Antibiotics in Ambulatory Care: Results from a Population-Based Randomized Controlled Trial." *Journal of Chronic Diseases* 40(5): 429-37.

Gonzales, R., K. K. Corbett, et al. (2005). "The 'Minimizing Antibiotic Resistance in Colorado' Project: Impact of Patient Education in Improving Antibiotic Use in Private Office Practices." *Health Services Research* 40(1): 101-116.

Gonzales, R., A. Sauaia, et al. (2004). "Antibiotic Treatment of Acute Respiratory Tract Infections in the Elderly: Effect of a Multidimensional Educational Intervention." *Journal of the American Geriatrics Society* 52(1): 39-45.

Gonzales, R., J. F. Steiner, et al. (1997). "Antibiotic Prescribing for Adults with Colds, Upper Respiratory Tract Infections, and Bronchitis by Ambulatory Care Physicians." *JAMA* 278(11): 901-4.

Gonzales, R., J. F. Steiner, et al. (1999). "Decreasing Antibiotic Use in Ambulatory Practice: Impact of a Multidimensional Intervention on the Treatment of Uncomplicated Acute Bronchitis in Adults." *JAMA* 281(16): 1512-1519.

Gonzales, R., J. F. Steiner, et al. (2001). "Impact of Reducing Antibiotic Prescribing for Acute Bronchitis on Patient Satisfaction." *Effective Clinical Practice* 4(3): 105-11.

Gross, P. A. and D. Pujat. (2001). "Implementing Practice Guidelines for Appropriate Antimicrobial Usage: A Systematic Review." *Medical Care* 39(8 Suppl 2): II55-69.

Guillemot, D., E. Varon, et al. (2005). "Reduction of Antibiotic Use in the Community Reduces the Rate of Colonization with Penicillin G-Nonsusceptible *Streptococcus pneumoniae.*" *Clinical Infectious Diseases* 41(7): 930-8.

Hillman, A. L., M. V. Pauly, et al. (1999). "Financial Incentives and Drug Spending in Managed Care." *Health Affairs* 18(2): 189-200.

Hoberman, A., D. P. Greenberg, et al. (2003). "Effectiveness of Inactivated Influenza Vaccine in Preventing Acute Otitis Media in Young Children: A Randomized Controlled Trial." *JAMA* 290(12): 1608-16.

Howard, D. H. (2005). "Life Expectancy and the Value of Early Detection." *Journal of Health Economics* 24(5): 891-906.

Huskamp, H. A., A. M. Epstein, et al. (2003). "The Impact of a National Prescription Drug Formulary on Prices, Market Share, and Spending: Lessons for Medicare?" *Health Affairs* 22(3): 149-158.

Huskamp, H. A., R. G. Frank, et al. (2005). "The Impact of a Three-Tier Formulary on Demand Response for Prescription Drugs." *Journal of Economics & Management Strategy* 14(3): 729-753.

Hutchinson, J. and R. Foley. (1997). *Influence of Nonmedical Factors on Antibiotic Prescription Rates.* Paper presented at the American Society of Microbiology (ASM) 37th Interscience Conference on Antimicrobial Agents and Chemotherapy. September 1997, Toronto, CA.

Jacobs, M. R. (2002). "Prevention of Otitis Media: Role of Pneumococcal Conjugate Vaccines in Reducing Incidence and Antibiotic Resistance." *The Journal of Pediatrics* 141(2): 287-293.

Johannes, L. (2005). "Choosing a Pill for That Cold." *The Wall Street Journal*, Dec. 27, D4.

Klugman, K. P. (2004). "Vaccination: A Novel Approach to Reduce Antibiotic Resistance." *Clinical Infectious Diseases* 39: 649-51.

Kumar, S., P. Little, et al. (2003). "Why Do General Practitioners Prescribe Antibiotics for Sore Throat? Grounded Theory Interview Study." *BMJ* 326(7381): 138.

Kyaw, M.H., R. Lynfield, et al. (2006). "Effect of Introduction of the Pneumococcal Conjugate Vaccine on Drug-Resistant *Streptococcus pneumoniae.*" *The New England Journal of Medicine* 354(14): 1455-63.

Laxminarayan, R. (2003). Economic Responses to the Problem of Drug Resistance. *The Resistance Phenomenon in Microbes and Infectious Disease Vectors: Implications for Human Health and Strategies for Containment—Workshop Summary.* Knobler, S. L., S. M. Lemon, et al. (eds). Washington, DC: National Academies Press, 121-129.

Laxminarayan, R. and M. L. Weitzman. (2002). "On the Implications of Endogenous Resistance to Medications." *Journal of Health Economics* 21(4): 709-718.

Leibowitz, A., W. G. Manning, et al. (1985). "The Demand for Prescription Drugs as a Function of Cost-Sharing." *Social Science & Medicine* 21(10): 251-277.

Little, P., K. Rumsby, et al. (2005). "Information Leaflet and Antibiotic Prescribing Strategies for Acute Lower Respiratory Tract Infection: A Randomized Controlled Trial." *JAMA* 293(24): 3029-35.

Macfarlane, J., W. Holmes, et al. (1997). "Influence of Patients' Expectations on Antibiotic Management of Acute Lower Respiratory Tract Illness in General Practice: Questionnaire Study." *BMJ* 315(7117): 1211-4.

Macfarlane, J., W. Holmes, et al. (2002). "Reducing Antibiotic Use for Acute Bronchitis in Primary Care: Blinded, Randomised Controlled Trial of Patient Information Leaflet." *BMJ* 324(7329): 91-94.

Mangione-Smith, R., E. A. McGlynn, et al. (1999). "The Relationship Between Perceived Parental Expectations and Pediatrician Antimicrobial Prescribing Behavior." *Pediatrics* 103(4 Pt 1): 711-8.

McCaig, L. F., R. E. Besser, et al. (2002). "Trends in Antimicrobial Prescribing Rates for Children and Adolescents." *JAMA* 287(23): 3096-102.

McCaig, L. F. and J. M. Hughes. (1995). "Trends in Antimicrobial Drug Prescribing Among Office-Based Physicians in the United States." *JAMA* 273(3): 214-9.

Metlay, J. P., J. A. Shea, et al. (2002). "Tensions in Antibiotic Prescribing: Pitting Social Concerns Against the Interests of Individual Patients." *Journal of General Internal Medicine* 17(2): 87-94.

Miller, G. E. and J. Hudson. (2006). "Children and Antibiotics: Analysis of Reduced Use, 1996-2001." *Medical Care* 44(5 Suppl): I36-I44.

Park, S., S. B. Soumerai, et al. (2005). "Antibiotic Use Following a Korean National Policy to Prohibit Medication Dispensing by Physicians." *Health Policy and Planning* 20(5): 302-9.

Paul, I. M., K. E. Yoder, et al. (2004). "Effect of Dextromethorphan, Diphenhydramine, and Placebo on Nocturnal Cough and Sleep Quality for Coughing Children and Their Parents." *Pediatrics* 114(1): e85-90.

Poehling, K. A., T. R. Talbot, et al. (2006). "Invasive Pneumococcal Disease Among Infants Before and After Introduction of Pneumococcal Conjugate Vaccine." *JAMA* 295(14): 1668-74.

Rabago, D., B. Barrett, et al. (2005). "Nasal Irrigation to Treat Acute Bacterial Rhinosinusitis." *American Family Physician* 72(9).

Rabago, D., A. Zgierska, et al. (2002). "Efficacy of Daily Hypertonic Saline Nasal Irrigation Among Patients with Sinusitis: A Randomized Controlled Trial." *The Journal of Family Practice* 51(12): 1049-55.

Ranji, S., M. Steinman, et al. (2006). *Antibiotic Prescribing Behavior.* Rockville, MD: Agency for Health care Research and Quality.

Rosenthal, M. B., R. G. Frank, et al. (2005). "Early Experience with Pay-For-Performance: From Concept to Practice." *JAMA* 294(14): 1788-93.

Roumie, C. L., N. B. Halasa, et al. (2005). "Trends in Antibiotic Prescribing for Adults in the United States—1995 to 2002." *Journal of General Internal Medicine* 20(8): 697-702.

Sbarbaro, J. A. (2001). "Can We Influence Prescribing Patterns?" *Clinical Infectious Diseases* 33 (Suppl 3): S240-4.

Schwartz, R. K., S. B. Soumerai, et al. (1989). "Physician Motivations for Nonscientific Drug Prescribing." *Social Science & Medicine* 28(6): 577-82.

Solomon, D. H., L. Van Houten, et al. (2001). "Academic Detailing to Improve Use of Broad-Spectrum Antibiotics at an Academic Medical Center." *Archives of Internal Medicine* 161(15): 1897-902.

Soumerai, S. B. and J. Avorn. (1990). "Principles of Educational Outreach ('Academic Detailing') to Improve Clinical Decision Making." *JAMA* 263(4): 549-56.

Steinke, D. T., T. M. MacDonald, et al. (1999). "The Doctor-Patient Relationship and Prescribing Patterns: A View from Primary Care." *Pharmacoeconomics* 16(6): 599-603.

Steinman, M. A., R. Gonzales, et al. (2003). "Changing Use of Antibiotics in Community-Based Outpatient Practice, 1991-1999." *Annals of Internal Medicine* 138(7): 525-33.

Stille, C. J., S. E. Andrade, et al. (2004). "Increased Use of Second-Generation Macrolide Antibiotics for Children in Nine Health Plans in the United States." *Pediatrics* 114(5): 1206-11.

Stivers, T. (2002a). "Participating in Decisions about Treatment: Overt Parent Pressure for Antibiotic Medication in Pediatric Encounters." *Social Science & Medicine* 54(7): 1111-30.

Stivers, T. (2002b). "Presenting the Problem in Pediatric Encounters: 'Symptoms Only' versus 'Candidate Diagnosis' Presentations." *Health Communication* 14(3): 299-338.

Sutter, A. I., M. Lemiengre, et al. (2003). "Antihistamines for the Common Cold." *Cochrane Database of Systematic Reviews* (3): CD001267.

Talbot, T. R., K. A. Poehling, et al. (2004). "Reduction in High Rates of Antibiotic-Nonsusceptible Invasive Pneumococcal Disease in Tennessee After Introduction of the Pneumococcal Conjugate Vaccine." *Clinical Infectious Diseases* 39(5): 641-8.

Tamblyn, R., R. Laprise, et al. (2001). "Adverse Events Associated With Prescription Drug Cost-Sharing Among Poor and Elderly Persons." *JAMA* 285(4): 421-429.

Taylor, J. A., T. S. C. Kwan-Gett, et al. (2003). "Effectiveness of an Educational Intervention in Modifying Parental Attitudes About Antibiotic Usage in Children." *Pediatrics* 111(5): e548-554.

Tomooka, L., C. Murphy, et al. (2000). "Clinical Study and Literature Review of Nasal Irrigation." *Laryngoscope* 110(7): 1189-93.

Vanden Eng, J., R. Marcus, et al. (2003). "Consumer Attitudes and Use of Antibiotics." *Emerging Infectious Diseases* 9(9): 1128-35.

Walter, L. C., N. P. Davidowitz, et al. (2004). "Pitfalls of Converting Practice Guidelines into Quality Measures: Lessons Learned From a VA Performance Measure." *JAMA* 291(20): 2466-70.

Whitney, C. G., M. M. Farley, et al. (2003). "Decline in Invasive Pneumococcal Disease after the Introduction of Protein-Polysaccharide Conjugate Vaccine." *The New England Journal of Medicine* 348(18): 1737-46.

Wu, J., D. Howard, et al. (2006). "Adherence to Infectious Disease Society of America Guidelines on Empiric Therapy for Patients with Community Acquired Pneumonia in a Commercially Insured Cohort." *Clinical Therapeutics* 28(9): 1451-61.

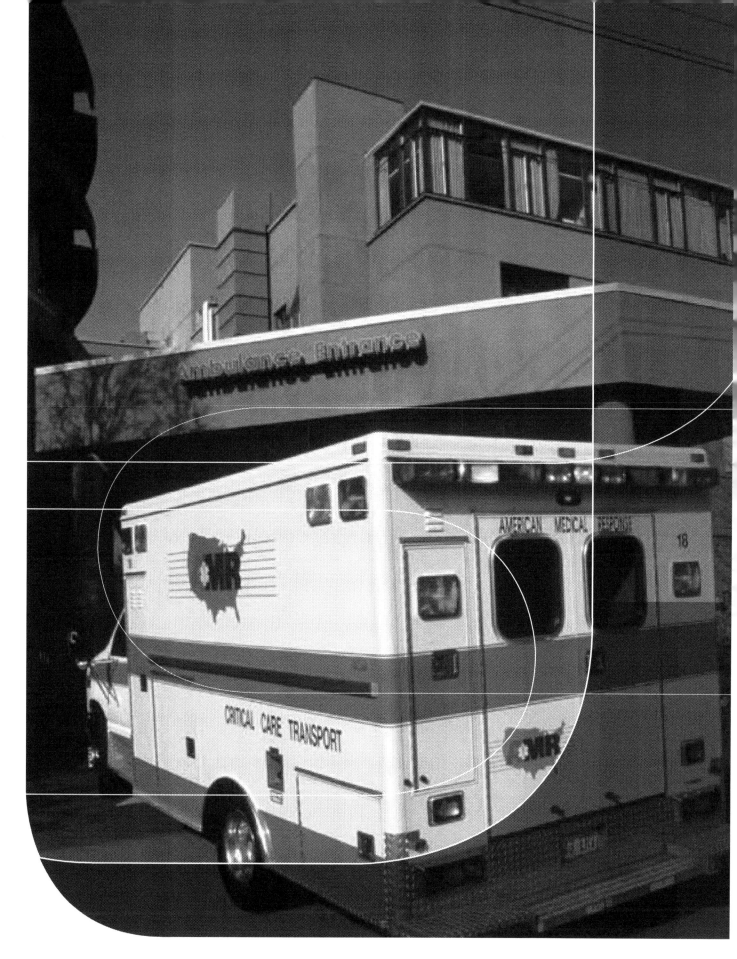

CHAPTER 4

# The role of **health care facilities**

*Ramanan Laxminarayan*

Rapid improvements in medical technology have made possible lifesaving interventions that keep hospitalized patients alive for longer. However, the downside of these interventions is that patients tend to be sicker, spend longer periods of time in the hospital, and are more in need of intensive medical care than before, leading to an increased prevalence of many nosocomial infections.[1] Also known as a hospital-acquired infection (HAI), a nosocomial infection is acquired in a hospital by a patient who was admitted for a reason other than that infection. Moreover, protracted illness and time on life support for these patients, many of whom are immuno-compromised, have increased reliance on antibiotics to help stave off infection, which in turn has resulted in increasing drug resistance among common, previously treatable HAIs.

According to the Centers for Disease Control and Prevention (CDC), HAIs account for an estimated 2 million infections and 90,000 deaths each year. Common HAIs include infections of surgical wounds, urinary tract infections, and lower respiratory tract infections. Infections acquired in health care institutions are among the top 10 causes of death in the United States: they are the primary cause of 1 percent of all deaths and are major contributors to an additional 2 percent of all deaths (Harrison and Lederberg 1998). Many of the endemic bacteria causing these infections are resistant to one or more classes of antibiotics' pose a major challenge to inpatient health, and significantly increase the costs of hospital stays. In fact, the United States has among the highest rates of drug-resistant hospital infections in the world, as described

---

1 Many of the procedures commonly performed on the seriously ill today, such as central venous catheterization and mechanical ventilation, predispose the patient to colonization with hospital-associated bacteria and an enhanced susceptibility to invasive infection with these agents.

in Chapter 1. Vancomycin-resistant enterococci (VRE) and methicillin-resistant *Staphylococcus aureus* (MRSA) are among the most important HAIs because they now account for a large fraction of nosocomial infections, but they are not the only problematic pathogens: increasingly, resistant Gram-negative bacteria such as *Pseudomonas aeruginosa* and *Klebsiella pneumoniae* are causing serious infections in hospital patients. Hospitals and long-term care facilities like nursing homes and hospice care tend to use large quantities of antibiotics and are consequently significant reservoirs of resistant pathogens. The ability of these pathogens to persist may be due to multiple interacting factors, including excessive antibiotic use, poor hygiene by health care workers, high susceptibility of patients, establishment in long-term care facilities (as well as in prisons and in the community), and colonization of hospital staff or the hospital environment. Each of these factors contributes to the emergence and establishment of endemicity within a clinical setting. In addition to the impact of endemic antibiotic-resistant bacteria on their own patients, hospitals are significant reservoirs of resistant pathogens that can be transported to other facilities.

Strategies for lowering the resistance levels in hospitals fall into three categories.[2] First is lowering antibiotic use by requiring preapproval for certain antibiotic prescriptions. Second is using creative antibiotic restriction strategies, such as cycling and treatment heterogeneity. Third is better infection control, which is applicable not just to resistant pathogens, but to all HAIs. Studies suggest that the economic and health benefits of many common interventions to lower the prevalence of HAIs exceed the costs. In this chapter we explore the incentives for hospitals[3] to invest in hospital infection control (HIC) and other measures to lower the

prevalence of resistant bacteria in their facilities, as well as potential regulatory solutions to encourage greater reporting and improved infection control.

■
## Economic costs and benefits

HAIs cost between $17 billion and $29 billion each year, and older studies have shown that a third of this burden can be lowered by adequate infection control programs (Haley, Culver et al. 1985). Numerous studies show that HAIs, especially resistant infections, cause longer hospital stays, greater risk of death, and much higher rates of hospitalization. There is also strong evidence that the overall economic benefits of infection control programs exceed costs by a wide margin and that "an effective infection control programme is one of the most cost-beneficial medical interventions available in modern public health" (Wenzel 1995). However, there is considerable disagreement over who bears the principal economic burden of these infections, and this influences incentives for health care facilities to engage in better infection control. In this section, we review existing evidence on the economic benefits of hospital infection control and incentives for hospitals to engage in it.

### :: COST OF HOSPITAL-ACQUIRED INFECTIONS

Numerous studies have documented the increased costs of nosocomial bloodstream infections, stretching back into the 1970s and 1980s. Pittet, Tarara et al. (1994) and Pittet and Wenzel (1995) found that during the 1980s, the incidence and risk of death from nosocomial bloodstream infections had risen markedly and that a patient with a nosocomial bloodstream infection was 35 percent more likely to die; for a patient who survived, extra costs attributable to the infection were approximately $40,000, and extra hospital costs, $6,000. Haley (1986) looked at all nosocomial infection costs and found that the average cost was about $1,800 per infection,

---

2   There are others, such as physician education, that are discussed in Chapter 3.

3   Although the problem of MRSA (and other HAIs) in nursing homes and prisons is not addressed in this chapter, a number of the recommendations made here are applicable to those situations as well.

with a maximum cost of about $42,000.

It is important to recognize the significant economic costs that nosocomial infections impose on both the hospital and the patient. The congressional Office of Technology Assessment has estimated the minimal hospital cost associated with nosocomial infections caused by antibiotic-resistant bacteria to be $1.3 billion per year (in 1992) (OTA 1995). This does not include the increased cost to patients, both monetarily and through the indirect and long-term morbidity and mortality consequences of resistant infections. In addition, most published studies have shown increased mortality risk on the order of 1.3 to 2 times, which may also have significant effects on indirect costs, such as long-term lost productivity. It is also important to understand that antibiotic resistance has an effect on many patients who do not become infected: they have to use stronger drugs, which may be more expensive, have more dangerous side effects, or be more toxic or possibly less effective than older or mainline drugs.

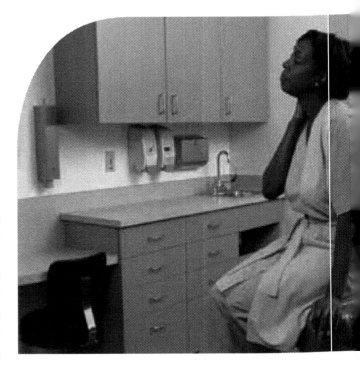

Those indirect costs aside, the cost of an antibiotic-resistant infection is still significant. According to Cosgrove, Qi et al. (2005), a nosocomial MRSA bacteremia significantly increases the length of hospital stays, the charges per patient, and hospital costs per case. They estimate that the excess cost of an MRSA bacteremia is $26,424 in patient charges and $14,655 in excess hospitals costs (total, $41,079 in excess charges) versus a control population. They also calculated costs for patients with methicillin-sensitive *Staphylococcus* infection (MSSA); these averaged $19,212 in excess patient charges and $10,655 in excess hospital costs (total, $29,867). McHugh and Riley (2004), similarly, estimated total per patient costs (as opposed to excess costs) of $9,699 for an MSSA infection versus $45,920 for an MRSA infection (an excess cost of $36,221).

Another important problem is surgical site infections, which are responsible for increased morbidity and mortality and cost hospitals more than $1.6 billion in extra charges each

year (Martone and Nichols 2001). Engemann, Carmeli et al. (2003) studied MRSA in surgical site infections in a large cohort at the Duke University Medical Center. MRSA in a surgical wound was found to result in more than a 12-fold increase in mortality versus non-infected patients and more than a 3-fold increase versus patients infected with MSSA. MRSA infections also cost patients about $40,000 more than an MSSA infection and about $84,000 more than an uninfected patient.

Vancomycin-resistant enterococci (VRE) are also associated with higher morbidity, mortality, and costs. Carmeli, Eliopoulos et al. (2002) found that a VRE infection led to longer hospital stays, a 2-fold increase in the rate of mortality, increased odds that a patient would require major surgery or be placed in the intensive care unit, and a 1.4-fold increase in hospital costs, which over the length of the study translated to excess costs of $2,974,478 (233 patients at an excess cost of

$12,766 each). In addition, the authors found an increase in the likelihood that a patient would end up being discharged to a long-term care facility, meaning that the additional costs of a VRE infection are significantly understated in the study and that they continue for many patients. These estimates are lower than in another study (Stosor, Peterson et al. 1998), which found that VRE bacteremia was associated with $27,190 in excess costs; yet another study (Song, Srinivasan et al. 2003) found mean excess costs of VRE to be $81,208.

> The average charge for a hospital admission in which a commercially insured patient contracted an infection was almost $258,000.

According to the Pennsylvania Health Care Cost Containment Council (PHC4) (PHC4 2005), the average charge for Pennsylvania Medicare patients with HAIs was about $160,000, five times the $32,000 average charge for Medicare patients who did not contract infections. Among Medicaid patients, the average charge was approximately $391,000 for patients who contracted infections while hospitalized, compared with an average of $29,700 when infections did not occur. Private commercial insurers of businesses and labor unions that provide health insurance were billed for almost 23 percent, or 2,633, of the reported hospital-acquired infections, which added $604 million in extra hospital charges. The average charge for a hospital admission in which a commercially insured patient contracted an infection was almost $258,000, compared with an average of $28,000 for admissions when infections did not occur. The average charge for stays in which uninsured patients contracted

infections reached almost $230,000, compared with $21,000 for an uninsured patient without an infection.

:: **BENEFITS OF HOSPITAL INFECTION CONTROL**

There has been relatively little evaluation of the impact of programs to lower antibiotic use within hospitals, but greater attention has been paid to the benefits and costs of infection control programs. For example, a program of intensive surveillance and interventions targeted at reducing the risk of hospital-acquired ventilator-associated pneumonia at the University of Massachusetts Medical Center in 1997–1998 lowered the incidence of this pneumonia and resulted in a cost savings greater than $350,000 (Lai, Baker et al. 2003).

Similarly, a 1994 VRE outbreak at the University of Virginia Hospital prompted an active surveillance program and contact isolation of colonized patients. The costs of the program, including time spent collecting samples, additional length of hospital stays in isolation, and laboratory fees, were estimated at $253,099 during the two-year study, during which time only one primary VRE bacteremia occurred (Muto, Giannetta et al. 2002). At a control hospital, where no such program was in place, there were 29 cases of VRE bacteremia during the corresponding period, and these resulted in an estimated cost of $761,320, based on an estimate of excess costs of $27,190 per case of VRE (Stosor, Peterson et al. 1998). Other per-case VRE cost estimates would value the program benefits at $357,448 (Carmeli, Eliopoulos et al. 2002) to $2,273,824 (Song, Srinivasan et al. 2003), but even the lower end of these benefits far exceeded the costs of the program.

Two Charleston, S.C., hospitals implemented an active surveillance program and a contact isolation protocol as recommended by the Society for Health care Epidemiology of America (SHEA). Based on prior rates of nosocomial infections, the new programs and protocols prevented an estimated 13 MRSA bacteremias and 9 surgical site infections for a cost savings of about $596,960 for the prevented bacteremias ($45,920 per case, based on McHugh and Riley 2004) and $756,000 for the prevented surgical site infections ($84,000 in excess costs per case, based on Engemann, Carmeli et al. 2003). The cost of implementing the program was $113,955, comprising $54,381 for surveillance and $59,574 for contact isolation (West, Guerry et al. 2006).

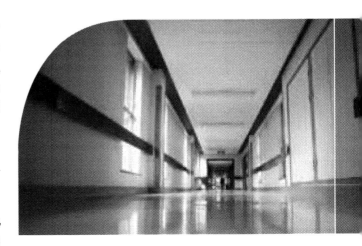

## Quality control in U.S. hospitals

This section provides an overview of how hospital quality, in general, and in particular with respect to infections, is currently measured and how hospitals are currently regulated or accredited.

### :: ACCREDITATION PROCESS

Hospital accreditation organizations such as the Joint Commission on Accreditation of Health care Organizations (JCAHO) currently do not require standards for antibiotic use, resistance, or nosocomial infections.[4] Hospitals are required to report only whether they follow a certain set of best practices for infection control, and not infection prevalence rates or resistance levels. JCAHO uses an on-site evaluation as the basis of accreditation. No long-term reporting is required for continued accreditation. Standards alone may not be able to solve the problem; a change in attitudes about hospital infections would come from a combination of education about the benefits of infection control and stronger incentives for hospitals to invest in control programs. Moreover, JCAHO clears more than 99 percent of all hospitals it inspects, which suggests that the current system is set up more to catch egregious violators of medical practices than to address pervasive problems like hospital-acquired infections and resistance (Gaul 2005).[5]

### :: HEALTH CARE QUALITY ORGANIZATIONS

The Leapfrog Consortium and other organizations that represent the interests of large purchasers of health care (such as automobile manufacturers) work with hospitals to encourage public reporting of health care quality and outcomes. They use a carrot-and-stick approach by rewarding hospitals that perform well and by leveraging consumer and health care purchaser choice to improve poor performers. Information on hospital infection control practices—including safety measures, hand washing, and vaccination of health care staff—is collected using self-reported surveys by hospitals. However, like JCAHO, Leapfrog may be better at separating good institutions from bad ones than at discerning finer indicators of performance, such as the prevalence of hospital-acquired infection.

In general, hospital-acquired infections and resistance are not a focus for existing organizations like JCAHO and Leapfrog. Although drug resistance can be seen as a quality issue, the current system for determining hospital quality may not work well to improve reporting or compliance with better infection control practices.

---

4 Based on a conversation with Dennis O'Leary, vice president, JCAHO, November 28, 2005.

5 In fact, concerns have been raised about the rigor of JCAHO's hospital surveys and its ability to catch even gross violations that have seriously compromised patient health.

## :: HICPAC AND SHEA GUIDELINES

Existing initiatives to improve hospital infection control—such as by CDC's Health care Infection Control Practices Advisory Committee (HICPAC) (McKibben, Horan et al. 2005) and SHEA (Muto, Jernigan et al. 2003)—provide guidance to hospitals to engage in greater infection control and thereby help prevent the spread of resistance. Both sets of guidelines are based on clinical evidence that the vast majority of MRSA and VRE infections are the result of transmission from patient to patient and not from *de novo* mutations, and thus they suggest that stringent infection control practices are probably the most important factor in limiting the spread of MRSA and VRE.

However, they differ in some important respects. In the context of MRSA and VRE, the SHEA guidelines call for active surveillance cultures to identify colonized patients, with barrier precautions for patients colonized or infected with MRSA and VRE. CDC guidelines, on the other hand, reject the need for active surveillance cultures on the grounds that they may impose unnecessary costs on hospitals. Nevertheless, the voluntary nature of these guidelines indicates that many hospitals are not likely to apply them unless they have a strong financial motivation for doing so.[6]

## :: REPORTING OF INFECTIONS AND RESISTANCE IN HOSPITALS

Since 1970, data on hospital infections and prevalence of MRSA and VRE (based on passive surveillance) have been voluntarily reported confidentially by hospitals participating in CDC's National Nosocomial Infection Surveillance (NNIS) program. These hospitals provide general medical-surgical inpatient services to adults or children requiring acute care. With a few exceptions, most current understanding of the extent of HAIs and drug resistance comes from the NNIS surveillance. However, there are important problems with this system that restrict its usefulness in delivering a comprehensive, nationwide picture of hospital infections and resistance. First, the nearly 300 hospitals that participate in the program are self-selected and represent only about 2 percent of hospitals, mainly academic centers—raising strong concerns about selection bias. Second, reporting within hospitals can change significantly. For instance, hospitals do not necessarily report data from the same intensive care unit each year, making comparisons across years problematic. Third, NNIS data are generally not available to researchers outside CDC because of confidentiality agreements signed with hospitals. This has restricted wider use of these data.

In recent years, under strong pressure from consumer advocates, some states have moved to require public reporting of hospital infections. In 2006, Consumers Union reported that six states (Illinois, Pennsylvania, Missouri, Florida, Virginia, and New York) had hospital infection disclosure laws, and 30

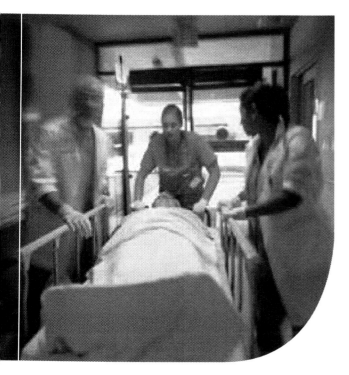

---

6   And, some hospitals do have such an incentive, as seen in studies reviewed earlier in this chapter.

states had introduced similar legislation requiring hospitals to report their infection levels to state monitoring bodies (CU 2006). By providing more transparency to consumers, better reporting of infection and resistance levels may give hospitals greater incentives to engage in infection control.

## Incentives and disincentives to control resistant HAIs

### :: HOSPITAL INCENTIVES

Despite some awareness of the problem and new measures to tackle the growing threat, the overall trend of infections, both susceptible and resistant, appears to be upward, as seen in Chapter 1. Antibiotic restrictions and better infection control are the two main tools available to hospitals. Currently, antibiotic restrictions are the main strategy reported by hospitals. Cost containment had been the original reason for implementing these restrictions (to divert physicians from expensive antibiotics to cheaper generics), but these reasons have been reborn in the form of concerns about drug resistance.

Programs intended to control antibiotic-resistant infections associated with health care have been around for a long time; however, implementation of these programs has been highly variable across facilities. Moreover, the guidelines have mostly focused on contact precautions that require staff hand washing, staff cohorting,[7] and use of protective equipment to prevent the spread of infection from patients identified as carrying an infection. Guidelines issued by SHEA in 2003, focused mainly on the spread of MRSA and VRE within the hospital setting, called existing measures insufficient and recommended active surveillance cultures to identify patients

colonized but not infected with resistant pathogens (Muto, Jernigan et al. 2003).

Next we consider important reasons why hospitals may not invest heavily in infection control programs on their own.

### :: HOSPITAL DISINCENTIVES

The extent to which hospitals bear the cost of resistant HAIs is a subject of disagreement, as is the extent to which these costs are passed on to Medicare, Medicaid, and private insurers. If reimbursement to the facility is tied to the number of days of hospitalization rather than by diagnosis-related group or episode of illness, the hospital may not bear any of the financial burden of extended hospital stays and may have few financial incentives for investing in HAIs even if the overall benefits of such investments exceed the costs.

A 1987 study that looked at charges associated with 9,423 nosocomial infections identified in 169,526 admissions, selected randomly from adult admissions to a random sample of U.S. hospitals, found that at least 95 percent of the cost savings obtained from preventing nosocomial infections represented financial gains to the hospital (Haley, White et al. 1987).

However, a series of recent reports from PHC4 find that Medicare and Medicaid bear the greatest burden of the additional cost of HAIs.[8] Pennsylvania hospitals billed the federal Medicare program and Pennsylvania's Medicaid program for 76 percent of the 11,668 hospital-acquired infections in 2004, with Medicare taking up much of the burden. The economic burden on government resources imposed by the additional hospital charges was estimated at $1 billion for Medicare and $372 million for Medicaid. Extrapolating from the figures in Pennsylvania to the entire country, PHC4 estimated that at least $20 billion was charged

---

7   This refers to assigning hospital staff to a limited number of patients rather than allowing for unlimited contact between health care workers and patients, which increases the likelihood of infection spread.

8   The PHC4 reports were based on a state law that required hospitals to submit data on some categories of HAIs to PHC4 starting January 2004. Starting January 1, 2006, nearly all hospital-acquired infections are reportable to PHC4 (PHC4 2006).

> Hospitals may actually benefit by extending the length of stay and may have fewer incentives to control infection levels within the hospital.

to Medicare to pay for HAIs during 2004. These figures indicate that hospitals may actually benefit by extending the length of stay and may have fewer incentives to control infection levels within the hospital.

Medicare is currently in the process of revising its rules on reimbursing for hospital-acquired infections, and these changes could have a significant impact on hospital incentives to invest in infection control. Some payers, such as Blue Cross–Blue Shield, have already made some payments contingent on lower rates of certain HAIs, and anecdotal evidence suggests that this has lowered the prevalence of those HAIs.

:: IMPACT OF LAWSUITS

Some hospitals have faced lawsuits from individual patients for HAIs, based on plaintiffs' claims that defendants (hospitals) failed to adhere to the standard of care for infection control.[9] A study from Philadelphia found that 72 percent of HAI malpractice cases in Philadelphia were either withdrawn or settled; when brought to trial, the plaintiff was more likely to prevail (Guinan, McGuckin et al. 2005). MRSA infections were the most common reason for lawsuits. Moreover,

MRSA in class I surgical sites were more likely to result in a victory for plaintiffs because national data show lower rates of infection for these surgeries, with the implication that these infections were preventable. The impact of lawsuits on infection control is unclear, but they may have made hospitals wary of reporting infection and resistance rates.

:: SHORT-TERM FINANCIAL CONSIDERATIONS

Even if most of the costs of HAIs can be passed on to payers, hospitals and long-term care facilities may bear at least some of the burden associated with the high cost of treating resistant infections. However, even for these limited costs, short-term cost considerations may trump the long-term gains of lower levels of resistance and infection for facilities in financial trouble. Are financially troubled institutions more likely to cut back on infection control? Do hospitals and long-term care facilities really behave optimally, or do they tend to be myopic because they fail to recognize the effect of resistance management and infection control on future costs? Also, to what extent are hospitals prompted by the threat of lawsuits to do a better job of controlling nosocomial infections and resistant pathogens? Answering these questions is pivotal to making policy decisions on how best to incentivize hospitals to invest in stronger infection control programs.

:: ISSUES OF AGENCY

Although the hospital as a whole may have an incentive to restrict the use of antibiotics and drug resistance, individual clinicians may not share the same incentives. Also, many physicians are not employees but consultants of hospitals and may therefore have a smaller incentive to care about costs imposed by resistance on hospitals. Conversely, the problem of resistance may be evident to infection control committees and clinicians, but they may not be able to convince senior management of the long-term financial benefits of lower levels of resistance. Management and operational structures of hospitals have implications both for investment in infection

---

9   Media reports of MRSA-related lawsuits are growing. In one recent example, the families of two women who died from MRSA infections while incarcerated at the jail in Allegheny County, Pennsylvania, sued the warden and other county officials for failing to provide medical care.

control and for implementation of control measures, but little is currently known about the influence of organizational culture and structure on infection and resistance levels.[10]

## :: INCENTIVES TO FREE-RIDE

Hospital infection control is expensive and becomes more difficult and less effective when patients enter the hospital already carrying the resistant pathogens. Recent research on incentives for hospitals to control HAIs suggests that the large spillovers of antibiotic-resistant bacteria among medical care facilities may be one factor that explains the lack of response (Smith, Levin et al. 2005). When institutions share patients, a person colonized in one facility may be responsible for introducing or increasing the prevalence of resistance in another facility.

Since any single hospital (especially in the current era of cost cutting and short-term financial pressures) may not see the benefits of its HIC program outside its own walls, hospitals may not benefit from decreasing the overall level of resistance in the catchment area when those patients are admitted later to other hospitals. Instead, hospitals may prefer to free-ride on the infection control investments of other hospitals. This results in an overall higher level of resistance.

Modeling shows that the selfishly "optimal" level of HIC that any hospital would undertake is lower the greater the number of hospitals that share a catchment area. In fact, it is in the interests of the hospital to spend less and free-ride on the efforts of other hospitals. When everyone free-rides, all hospitals will spend less on HIC, leading to epidemics that develop earlier and faster. A much better outcome can be

achieved through regulation and the resulting coordination between facilities.

A good example comes from the Siouxland experience. An epidemic of VRE in the Siouxland region of Iowa, Nebraska, and South Dakota was first detected in late 1996. Within a short time, VRE had quickly spread to nearly half of the health care facilities in the region. In response, a VRE task force was constituted with representatives from acute care and long-term care facilities and public health departments in the region (Ostrowsky, Tricke et al. 2001). Following a comprehensive two-year intervention (including aggressive culturing to identify VRE-colonized patients, isolation of patients, improved antibiotic use, sterile device measures, improved staff hand hygiene, and sharing of information

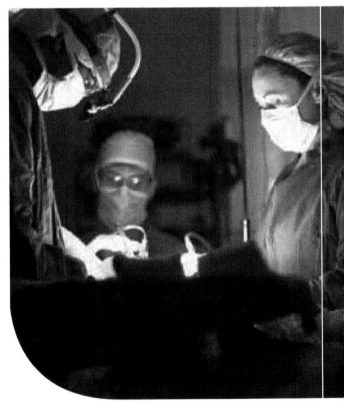

---

10   Hospital objectives may be multifaceted. Many participants at our consultations agreed that although hospital managers care about reducing infection-related mortality, they are less adept at seeing the long-term health and economic benefits of infection control. Some of the short-sightedness is reflected in compensation of infectious disease clinicians and nurses: an infection control nurse typically earns less than a bedside nurse and consequently there is a shortage in supply.

BOX 4.1

## THE DUTCH EXPERIENCE WITH CONTROLLING MRSA

MRSA incidence rates in the Netherlands are among the lowest in the world—1.1 percent—in contrast to more than 25 percent in France, Spain, and Belgium and 43.5 percent in the United Kingdom (The National Institute for Public Health and the Environment (RIVM)) (see Figure 1.4). This extremely low rate is attributable to a decade-old national "search and destroy" policy to limit the spread of MRSA. The implementing guidelines are based on the premise that the best way to fight MRSA is to identify it as early as possible and to isolate infected or possibly infected patients. Patients and health care workers are categorized according to risk and screened regularly based on those risk assessments. For example, all patients treated in a foreign hospital are considered at high risk of being MRSA carriers and thus are isolated until cultures prove negative (Dutch Workingparty Infection Prevention 2005). Most importantly, the policy requires the cooperation of all health care facilities and is enforced by the Dutch government.

The policy has not been cheap to implement. Over the course of 10 years, the MRSA policy resulted in more than 2,265 lost hospitalization days (Vriens, Blok et al. 2002). Wards had to be closed 48 times, 29 health care workers had to temporarily discontinue working, and 78,000 additional cultures had to be performed. However, it is estimated that the 6 million euros realized as benefits of the campaign in terms of averted MRSA infections and increased vancomycin-resistance in other bacteria (*S. aureus* and VRE) far outweighed the cost (2.8 million euros) of hospital infection control in the Netherlands during the period.

A new strain of MRSA appeared in 1999 but was not immediately recognized as such because of the limited sensitivity of the tests at the time. Within weeks this new strain, still unrecognized, had spread to several health care facilities. By increasing the sensitivity of the tests and maintaining intensive screening of both patients and health care workers, by the end of 2003, the new strain of MRSA was under control (Vos, Ott et al. 2005). Controlling the spreading epidemic was possible only because of the national strategy: if any hospital had lapsed, MRSA would spread to all the other institutions fairly quickly.

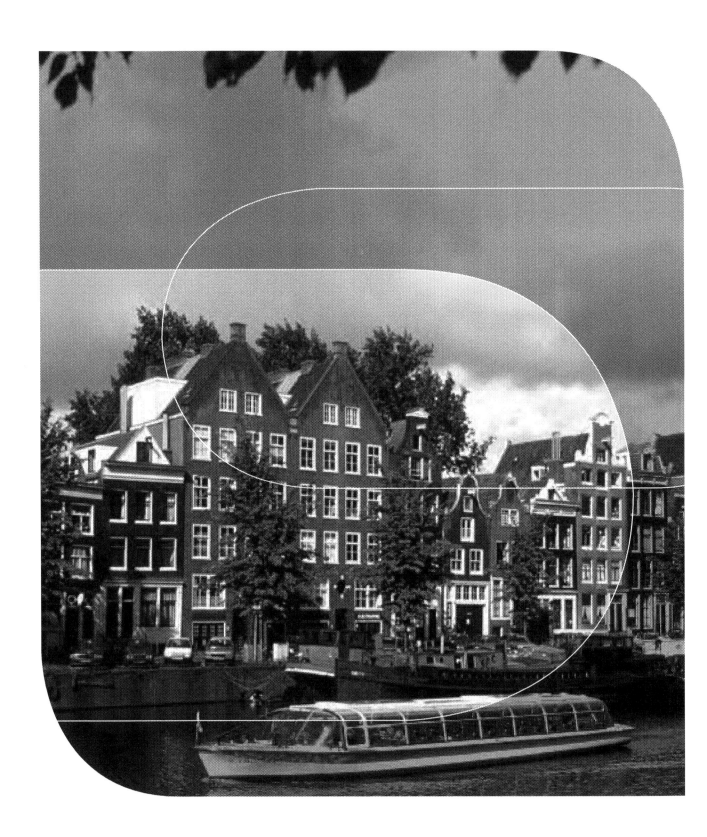

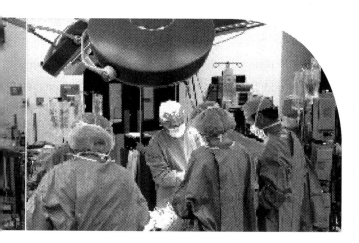

among institutions), VRE was eliminated from all acute care facilities and significantly reduced in long-term care facilities in the region. This could not have happened without coordination. When hospitals are unwilling to coordinate on their own, regulation will ensure that no single hospital free-rides on the efforts of others. Regulations that require portability of patient records (which could show which patients are colonized) could help hospitals in identifying high-risk carriers of resistant pathogens.

The similarly successful experience of Dutch hospitals in lowering the prevalence of MRSA is described in Box 4.1.

:: INCENTIVES TO REPORT INFECTION LEVELS

Hospitals have a clear incentive to downplay infection levels in their facilities, since accurate reporting could decrease demand for their services. "Report cards" that provide patients with information on hospital quality, including nosocomial infection rates, may encourage hospitals to discriminate against sicker patients or those coming from long-term care facilities because they might be more likely to carry a resistant pathogen.[11] To address this problem,

Florida and some other states that publicly report outcome indicators by hospital risk adjust the data to account for the fact that some hospitals admit more patients who are sicker and require more resources than the average patient. An alternative strategy would be to monitor and subsidize inputs for hospital infection control rather than monitoring the outputs—that is, infection levels. Educational efforts to get hospitals to recognize the long-term gains of infection control may also be part of the solution.

Hospital report cards also should be issued by an independent agency that is less susceptible to political pressure. These reports, if issued by government agencies, can be influenced or quashed by interference from the governor or state senators, who in turn are influenced by campaign contributions from wealthy doctors. Governmental policy can also influence the timing of the release of reports.

Some degree of enforcement is required, via periodic external surveillance cultures, withdrawal of approval for state Medicare reimbursement, or fines. Because reporting requirements can create perverse incentives—for example, hospitals that suspect high levels of resistance may cut back on surveillance expenditures—any reporting program needs to be designed to take these factors into consideration.

## Recommendations

Hospitals are an important reservoir for resistant pathogens, and the problem of resistant infections is emblematic of broader problems with ensuring health care quality. The issue is not knowing how to address resistant infections in hospitals[12]—good examples exist, from both the United

---

11  A related study in the context of cardiac surgery found that the use of hospital report cards in New York and Pennsylvania led to improved

matching of patients with hospitals, but also gave doctors and hospitals an incentive to turn away severely ill patients who were more difficult to treat. This resulted in higher levels of resource use and worse health outcomes, particularly for sicker patients (Dranove, Kessler et al. 2002).

12  Although much of the problem with drug resistance in hospitals

States and abroad, of how to maintain low levels of resistance in health care settings—but rather, understanding why some facilities have an incentive to invest in these programs while others do not.

Regulatory agencies play two important roles in the antibiotic resistance problem. One is to enable cooperative outcomes better than those attained if hospitals behave in their own self-interest. Regional coordination in infection control efforts may be one of several solutions to this dilemma (Kaye, Engemann et al. 2006). Another is to make public the data on resistance and infection levels so that hospitals have an incentive to invest in addressing the problem. Here we propose ways to encourage reporting and control of resistant infections and improve surveillance, and we also recommend additional research.

■

## Conclusions

1.  Hospital reimbursement policies for HAIs could be linked to levels of infection and drug resistance. Tying Medicare and private insurance payments to a hospital to its levels of infection control may be one approach.

2.  Subsidizing inputs for infection control and surveillance programs would provide a greater incentive for hospitals to invest in them. Chapter 6, on health insurance and Medicare, describes such a program.

3.  State requirements for reporting of hospital infections should adjust the data for risk so that hospitals that admit sicker patients are not penalized for having higher levels of antibiotic use and infection.

4.  The national hospital infection and resistance surveillance system should be more comprehensive. Ideally, it would be separate from JCAHO and other accreditation groups and would take the approach used by several states: it would collect nationwide data not just on outcomes (infections and resistance) but also on inputs, such as antibiotic use, number of infection control nurses, and physical inputs for HIC. Given the incentive problems with reporting outcomes, independent monitoring and reporting of infections should be complemented with reports on infection control inputs.

5.  Legal avenues for responding to resistance should be examined, perhaps involving a combination of workplace safety and labor laws (e.g., penalizing hospitals for a failure to protect nursing staff if they are at risk). Studies indicate that nurses are at-risk for infections caused by *C. difficile* and *E. coli*, however this risk is believed to be low (Sepkowitz 1996a; 1996b).

6.  Research needs to address the important policy-relevant questions. Little is known about the institutional characteristics (ownership structure,[13] proximity to other hospitals and facilities) that predict resistance. We also know little about the costs of surveillance and infection control for a typical hospital and how these compare with other hospital expenses. Additional data will help determine the burden of infection control on hospital budgets and inform the design of taxes and subsidies for specific inputs for infection control.

7.  A policy research program is needed to explore how to create incentives for hospitals to conduct surveillance and reporting, not just of infections but also of other important health care quality measures.

---

is related to lack of sufficient infection control rather than to excessive antibiotic use, hospitals have tended to focus on the antibiotic use issue to a greater extent. Some hospitals have pursued cycling and other antibiotic restriction policies even though ecologists have questioned the soundness of these strategies (Bergstrom, Lo et al. 2004).

---

13  Categories include government hospitals, for-profit hospitals, nonprofit teaching hospitals, and nonprofit nonacademic hospitals.

# References

Bergstrom, C. T., M. Lo, et al. (2004). "Ecological Theory Suggests that Antimicrobial Cycling Will Not Reduce Antimicrobial Resistance in Hospitals." *Proceedings of the National Academy of Sciences of the United States of America* 101(36): 13285-90.

Carmeli, Y., G. Eliopoulos, et al. (2002). "Health and Economic Outcomes of Vancomycin-Resistant Enterococci." *Archives of Internal Medicine* 162(19): 2223-2228.

Cosgrove, S. E., Y. Qi, et al. (2005). "The Impact of Methicillin Resistance in *Staphylococcus aureus* Bacteremia on Patient Outcomes: Mortality, Length of Stay, and Hospital Charges." *Infection Control and Hospital Epidemiology* 26: 166-174.

CU. (2006). http://www.consumersunion.org (accessed October 18, 2006). Consumers Union.

Dranove, D., D. P. Kessler, et al. (2002). "Is More Information Better? The Effects of 'Report Cards' on Health Care Providers." Working paper W8697. Cambridge, MA: NBER (National Bureau of Economic Research).

Engemann, J. J., Y. Carmeli, et al. (2003). "Adverse Clinical and Economic Outcomes Attributable to Methicillin Resistance among Patients with *Staphylococcus aureus* Surgical Site Infection." *Clinical Infectious Diseases* 36: 592-598.

Gaul, G. M. (2005). "Accreditors Blamed for Overlooking Problems: Conflict of Interest Cited Between Health Facilities, Group That Assesses Conditions." *Washington Post*. Washington, DC, July 25, A01.

Guinan, J. L., M. McGuckin, et al. (2005). "A Descriptive Review of Malpractice Claims for Health Care-Acquired Infections in Philadelphia." *American Journal of Infection Control* 33(5): 310-2.

Haley, R.W. (1986). *Managing Hospital Infection Control for Cost Effectiveness: A Strategy for Reducing Infectious Complications.* Chicago: American Hospital Publishing, Inc.

Haley, R. W., D. H. Culver, et al. (1985). "The Efficacy of Infection Surveillance and Control Programs in Preventing Nosocomial Infections in US Hospitals." *American Journal of Epidemiology* 121(2): 182-205.

Haley, R. W., J. W. White, et al. (1987). "The Financial Incentive for Hospitals to Prevent Nosocomial Infections under the Prospective Payment System. An Empirical Determination from a Nationally Representative Sample." *JAMA* 257(12): 1611-4.

Harrison, P. F. and J. Lederberg (eds.). (1998). *Antimicrobial Resistance: Issues and Options, Workshop Report.* Forum on Emerging Infections. Washington, DC: Institute of Medicine.

Jevons, M. (1961). "Celbenin-Resistant Staphylococci." *BMJ* 1: 124-5.

Kaye, K. S., J. J. Engemann, et al. (2006). "Favorable Impact of an Infection Control Network on Nosocomial Infection Rates in Community Hospitals." *Infection Control and Hospital Epidemiology* 27(3): 228-32.

Lai, K. K., S. P. Baker, et al. (2003). "Impact of a Program of Intensive Surveillance and Interventions Targeting Ventilated Patients in the Reduction of Ventilator-Associated Pneumonia and Its Cost-Effectiveness." *Infection Control and Hospital Epidemiology* 24(11): 859-863.

Laxminarayan, R., D. L. Smith, et al. (2005). "On the Importance of Incentives in Hospital Infection Control Spending." *Discovery Medicine* 5(27): 303-308.

Martone, W. J. and R. L. Nichols. (2001). "Recognition, Prevention, Surveillance, and Management of Surgical Site Infections: Introduction to the Problem and Symposium Overview." *Clinical Infectious Diseases* 33: S67-S68.

McHugh, C. G. and L. W. Riley. (2004). "Risk Factors and Costs Associated With Methicillin-Resistant *Staphylococcus aureus* Bloodstream Infections." *Infection Control and Hospital Epidemiology* 25(5): 425-430.

McKibben, L., T. Horan, et al. (2005). "Guidance on Public Reporting of Health care-Associated Infections: Recommendations of the Health care Infection Control Practices Advisory Committee." *American Journal of Infection Control* 33(4): 217-26.

Muto, C. A., E. T. Giannetta, et al. (2002). "Cost-Effectiveness of Perirectal Surveillance Cultures for Controlling Vancomycin-Resistant Enterococcus." *Infection Control and Hospital Epidemiology* 23(8): 429-435.

Muto, C. A., J. A. Jernigan, et al. (2003). "SHEA Guideline for Preventing Nosocomial Transmission of Multidrug-Resistant Strains of *Staphylococcus aureus* and Enterococcus." *Infection Control and Hospital Epidemiology* 24(5): 362-386.

Ostrowsky, B. E., W. E. Trick, et al. (2001). "Control of Vancomycin-Resistant Enterococcus in Health Care Facilities in a Region." *The New England Journal of Medicine* 344(19): 1427-1433.

OTA. (1995). *Impact of Antibiotic-Resistant Bacteria: A Report to the U.S. Congress*. Washington, DC: Government Printing Office. Office of Technology Assessment.

PHC4. (2005). "Reducing Hospital-Acquired Infections: The Business Case." Research Brief No. 8. http://www.phc4.org/reports/ researchbriefs/111705/docs/researchbrief2005report_ hospacqinfections_bizcase.pdf (accessed March 5, 2007). Pennsylvania Health Care Cost Containment Council.

PHC4. (2006). *Hospital-acquired Infections in Pennsylvania 2005*. http:// www.phc4.org/reports/hai/05/default.htm (accessed December 11, 2006). Pennsylvania Health Care Cost Containment Council.

Pittet, D., D. Tarara, et al. (1994). "Nosocomial Bloodstream Infection in Critically Ill Patients. Excess Length of Stay, Extra Costs, and Attributable Mortality." *JAMA* 271(20): 1598-1601.

Pittet, D. and R. P. Wenzel. (1995). "Nosocomial Bloodstream Infections. Secular Trends in Rates, Mortality, and Contribution to Total Hospital Deaths." *Archives of Internal Medicine* 155(11): 1177-1184.

RIVM. (2005). "European Antimicrobial Resistance Surveillance System (EARSS)." http://www.rivm.nl/earss/ (accessed on January 18, 2005). The National Institute for Public Health and the Environment.

Sepkowitz, K.A. (1996a). "Occupationally Acquired Infections in Health Care Workers: Part I." *Annals of Internal Medicine* 125(10): 826-834.

Sepkowitz, K.A. (1996b). "Occupationally Acquired Infections in Health Care Workers: Part II." *Annals of Internal Medicine* 125(11): 917-928.

Smith, D. L., S. A. Levin, et al. (2005). "Strategic Interactions in Multi-Institutional Epidemics of Antibiotic Resistance." *Proceedings of the National Academy of Sciences of the United States of America* 102(8): 3153-8.

Sohn, A. H., B. E. Ostrowsky, et al. (2001). "Evaluation of a Successful Vancomycin-Resistant Enterococcus Prevention Intervention in a Community of Health Care Facilities." *American Journal of Infection Control* 29(1): 53-57.

Song, X., A. Srinivasan, et al. (2003). "Effect of Nosocomial Vancomycin-Resistant Enterococcal Bacteremia on Mortality, Length of Stay, and Costs." *Infection Control and Hospital Epidemiology* 24(4): 251-256.

Stosor, V., L. R. Peterson, et al. (1998). "*Enterococcus faecium* Bacteremia: Does Vancomycin Resistance Make a Difference?" *Archives of Internal Medicine* 158(5): 522-527.

Vos, M. C., A. Ott, et al. (2005). "Successful Search-and-Destroy Policy for Methicillin-Resistant *Staphylococcus aureus* in The Netherlands." *Journal of Clinical Microbiology* 43(4): 2034-2035.

Vriens, M., H. Blok, et al. (2002). "Costs Associated with a Strict Policy to Eradicate Methicillin-Resistant *Staphylococcus aureus* in a Dutch University Medical Center: A 10-Year Survey." *European Journal of Clinical Microbiology and Infectious Diseases* 21(11): 782-786.

Wagenvoort, J. H. (2000). "Dutch Measures to Control MRSA and the Expanding European Union." *Euro Surveillance* 5(3): 26-28.

Wenzel, R. P. (1995). "The Lowbury Lecture. The Economics of Nosocomial Infections." *The Journal of Hospital Infection* 31(2): 79-87.

West, T. E., C. Guerry, et al. (2006). "Effect of Targeted Surveillance for Control of Methicillin-Resistant *Staphylococcus aureus* in a Community Hospital System." *Infection Control and Hospital Epidemiology* 27(3): 233-238.

WIP. (2005). Policy for Methicillian-resistant *Staphylococcus aureus*. http://www.wip.nl (accessed May 31, 2006). Dutch Workingparty Infection Prevention.

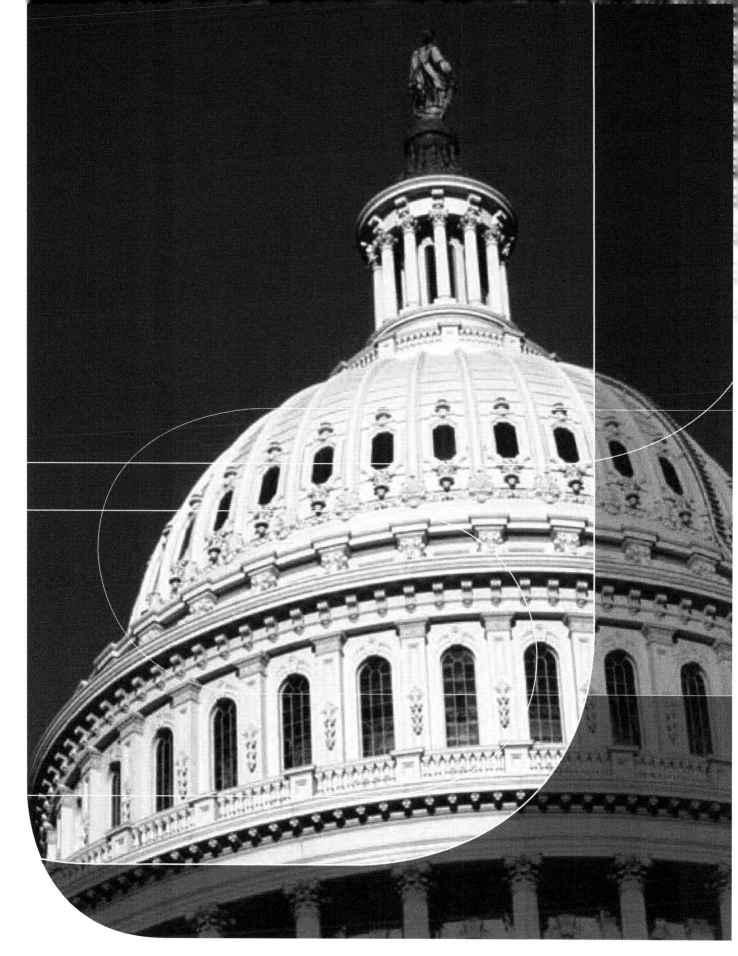

C H A P T E R

# 5

# The role of the **federal government**

*Ramanan Laxminarayan*

Earlier chapters have described the externalities generated by antibiotic overuse and insufficient infection control and have made the case for why individual actors (including patients, physicians, and hospital administrators) may lack sufficient incentives to manage for resistance. In the absence of our ability to assign strict liability for antibiotic overuse or lack of infection control to those different actors, the market failure evident in the negative externalities provides a strong rationale for government involvement to ensure that antibiotics are produced and used in a sustainable manner.

There is a role for both federal and state agencies to act on the antibiotic resistance problem; this chapter focuses on the former. The Centers for Disease Control and Prevention (CDC), the Food and Drug Administration (FDA), and the National Institutes of Health (NIH) are already engaged in a response to the resistance problem. CDC has been promoting campaigns to lower antibiotic use in hospitals and outpatient settings; FDA has acted to introduce labeling on antibiotics to warn consumers of the emergence of drug resistance, and has disallowed the use of antibiotics in animals in an instance where there was a likely threat to human health; and NIH has diverted modest funding to support discovery of new antibiotics. However, no single

government agency currently has the ability or resources to respond adequately to the threat of antibiotic resistance.

Since 2001, recognizing the need for a coordinated response to the problem, a number of federal agencies, under the leadership of CDC, NIH, and FDA, have operated under the auspices of the Interagency Task Force on Antimicrobial Resistance (ITFAR).[1] The action plan drafted by the task

---

1    The task force also includes representatives from the Agency for Health care Research and Quality, the Centers for Medicare and Medicaid Services (formerly the Health Care Financing Administration), the Department of Agriculture, the Department of Defense, the Department of Veterans Affairs, the Environmental Protection Agency, and the Health Resources and Services Administration.

force describes specific, coordinated actions to be undertaken by federal agencies covering a range of issues—from better lab standards for resistant pathogens to educational interventions for helping physicians with appropriate antibiotic prescribing. Several action items on the plan also relate to economic incentives, specifically removing barriers to the use of diagnostics in clinical care settings and improving incentives for new drug development. In this chapter we examine possible roles for the federal government in addressing some of the externalities implicit in the antibiotic resistance problem.

------

## What government can do

An important reason for government involvement in antibiotic resistance is that antibiotic effectiveness is a common property resource. In this regard, it shares features with other resources, such as forests or fish, where excluding users may be difficult and the potential for overexploitation is serious; hence federal agencies, such as the Forest Service or the National Oceanic and Atmospheric Administration have a clear management role. There is a long documented history of successes and failures in the management of common property resources that efforts to manage antibiotic effectiveness can draw from. A fundamental challenge of managing resources is to find the appropriate mix of policies that alter incentives for individual decisionmakers to consider the effect of their actions on everyone else, and policies that call for oversight and action by government agencies.[2]

An important distinction in the case of antibiotics is that the drugs themselves are developed and sold by private economic agents, but this does not preclude Congress from acting to help sustain the effectiveness of antibiotics. Federal law gives CDC, NIH, and FDA clearly defined and separate roles in

------

2   Both types of policies are challenging to implement in the context of medical practice, for reasons we discuss later.

# A stronger mandate and funding to improve surveillance for drug resistance is an important first step.

addressing public health problems, and these agencies can work on the following three objectives as appropriate to their missions: 1) improving the quality of antibiotic use, 2) improving hospital infection control to prevent emergence and transmission of resistant pathogens, and 3) improving the supply of new antibiotics.

### :: IMPROVING ANTIBIOTIC USE

The two federal agencies that are best positioned to help improve the quality of antibiotic use are CDC and FDA. CDC is charged, broadly speaking, with surveillance and response to epidemics and disease outbreaks. This gives CDC a mandate to work, largely in a technical advisory capacity, to prevent the emergence of drug resistance and to be actively involved in containing outbreaks of resistant pathogens. Surveillance for antibiotic resistance in both hospitals and communities is already an important function. However, CDC cannot require hospitals to report resistance levels, and under its current arrangements it cannot publicly release any disaggregated data on hospital infection or resistance levels. A stronger mandate and funding to improve surveillance for drug resistance is an important first step.

Another useful role for CDC is educating physicians about the dangers of drug resistance and the importance of appropriate prescribing, even though educational measures go only so far in changing behavior. CDC can also pay for research to improve the use of antibiotics in hospital and outpatient settings; in fact, it has done so in the past (to evaluate the use of antibiotic cycling programs to delay the emergence of resistance), although the quantity of such funding has been quite small.

CDC's strongest role is in influencing clinical practice based on a broader, multidisciplinary view of resistance, rather than just through a biomedical lens. For example, CDC could take the lead in integrating ecological understanding into antibiotic use and promote fundamental change in our thinking, including a rethinking of clinical guidelines for antibiotics. Current guidelines encourage the use of the least expensive or most cost-effective antibiotics, and thus a small number of antibiotics are prescribed extensively. Ecological theory, however, suggests that this practice may promote the development of resistance much more rapidly than if a diverse set of antibiotics were used. Moreover, treatment guidelines that call for "conserving" some antibiotics for infections that are not treatable by less expensive drugs inadvertently create disincentives for research and development efforts on new antibiotics (see Chapter 7).

FDA can regulate antibiotic use in the interests of patient safety. It has done so in the context of drug resistance in two instances. In 2000, FDA intervened to require two pharmaceutical companies to stop selling fluoroquinolones for growth promotion in poultry because of concerns that this was causing drug-resistant *Campylobacter* infections in humans (Box 5.1). In 2003, FDA issued new labeling regulations designed to help slow the development of drug-resistant bacterial strains by reducing the inappropriate prescription of antibiotics to children and adults for such common ailments as ear infections and chronic coughs.[3]

---

3  FDA can also require testing after approval of fast-track drugs but has no enforcement power, so this approach is infrequently taken. In addition, it is unclear what mandate FDA has to even regulate drugs once they have been approved. There is certainly no organizational motivation or structure in place to do this.

:: **IMPROVING INFECTION CONTROL IN HOSPITALS**

CDC has a public health mandate to address hospital-acquired infections (HAIs) whether or not they are drug resistant. CDC may be better positioned to respond to public health emergencies caused by an outbreak of resistant pathogens, however, than to encourage hospitals to take long-term measures to contain drug resistance. The largely advisory and educational role that CDC can play in ensuring hospital infection control and judicious antibiotic use (except perhaps in a time of crisis) has constrained a strong federal response to the problem. However, CDC may be able to change incentives for private providers and hospitals to invest more strongly in infection control.

For instance, CDC can promote the use of regional cooperatives between hospitals to ensure that efforts to control HAIs are coordinated at a regional scale rather than at the scale of a single hospital. As discussed in Chapter 4, an individual hospital may have little incentive to invest in HAIs if it admits patients colonized at other facilities that have poor infection control measures. The "commons" problem associated with HAIs can be addressed by state-level health authorities but with a coordinating function played by CDC.

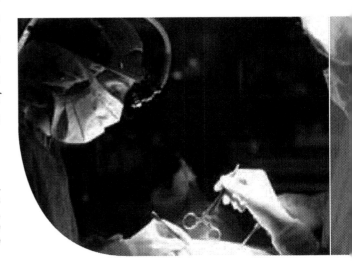

**BOX 5.1**

# REGULATING BAYTRIL: INCENTIVES FOR BAYER

In 2000, FDA announced that the proportion of *Campylobacter* infections resistant to fluoroquinolones—a powerful class of antibiotics for use in human treatment and for growth promotion—had increased significantly since one type of the drug, enrofloxacin, had been approved for use in poultry in the United States. Over growing concerns about the impact of this use on human health, FDA withdrew permission for Bayer to sell Baytril, their enrofloxacin product, for growth promotion. It was only after a lengthy court battle that ended in 2005, however, that Bayer finally agreed to comply with FDA's ruling. One would have expected Bayer to be concerned about the impact of resistance on demand for Cipro (which belongs to the same class of antibiotics as Baytril), its highly successful fluoroquinolone sold for human use.

Although the quantity of antibiotics sold for growth promotion is large, the economic value of this market to antibiotics producers is much smaller than that for human antibiotics, which sell at a higher price. For instance, in 2000, Bayer's sales of Cipro (the brand name of ciprofloxacin) amounted to roughly 1.8 billion euros, compared with only 170 million euros for sales of Baytril. Why would firms acting in their own self-interest jeopardize their profitable human drugs market to retain a much smaller market for growth-promoting agricultural drugs? After all, if firms fully internalized the consequences of future resistance, then there would be no need for regulatory intervention to protect the future effectiveness of these valuable drugs.

One answer is that there may be market failure. Often, many firms make different antibiotics that are derivatives of the same basic chemical entity. For instance, there are currently at least four firms that make fluoroquinolones. Because the resource embodied in the effectiveness of a class of antibiotics is available to several pharmaceutical firms, no single firm has incentive to take into full consideration the effect of its sales of antibiotics on future antibiotic effectiveness—even though resistance may be an inevitable consequence of antibiotic use.

Another major reason is patent expiration. Pharmaceutical companies have an incentive to sell as much of a drug as possible before their patent expires and generics enter the market. They may be much less concerned about engendering resistance to their products. In the case of Bayer, Cipro and Baytril were scheduled to go off-patent in 2004 and 2006, respectively. Thus, Bayer correctly predicted that their sales of Cipro would dramatically fall after going off-patent (sales dropped to 525 million euros in 2005). Since Baytril use had little effect on resistance, sales, and profits of Cipro in the short term, Bayer had no incentive to stop selling the drug. Instead, Bayer had an incentive to fight the FDA ruling since Baytril recorded more than a billion euros in sales between 2000 and 2005.

Antibiotic effectiveness is a common property resource, and the classic externality problem arises when, from a societal perspective, too many doses of antibiotics are sold. From an economic perspective, the price of antibiotics sold for growth promotion may not adequately reflect the true social cost of resistance associated with such use, and it is likely that sales of antibiotics for growth promotion in food animals would decline if farmers and pharmaceutical companies faced the full resistance-related costs.

CDC can conduct surveillance and set guidelines but may be more constrained from the standpoint of enforcement. The Centers for Medicare and Medicaid Services in the Department of Health and Human Services can help provide incentives by tying Medicare and Medicaid reimbursements to physician antibiotic prescribing and hospital infection control practices; this is discussed in greater detail in Chapter 6.

:: IMPROVING THE SUPPLY OF NEW ANTIBIOTICS

Development of new antibiotics appears to be on the decline. According to a recent review, FDA approval of new antibacterial agents decreased by 56 percent between the periods 1983–1987 and 1998–2002 (Spellberg, Powers et al. 2004). Only 6 of 506 drugs disclosed in the developmental programs of the largest pharmaceutical and biotechnology companies are antibacterial agents, and all of these new drugs belong to existing classes of antibiotics.

NIH and FDA are positioned to act to improve the supply of new antibiotics (Chapter 7). The National Institute of Allergy and Infectious Diseases, one of the largest institutes of NIH, has funded work on the basic biology of resistant organisms as well as applied research on new diagnostic techniques, therapies, and preventive measures. NIH support for basic research is an important subsidy to drug development and should be continued. NIH can lower the cost of product development by paying for basic scientific research to identify new target organisms and drugs that can work on these targets.[4]

FDA's role in new drug development is more complex, since it must ensure the safety and efficacy of new antibiotics without discouraging new drugs. FDA currently requires that manufacturers of new antibiotic demonstrate that their medications are noninferior to currently available antimicrobials. Some have argued that this places a heavy burden on new antibiotic development and has discouraged

> Faster approvals may be less desirable than direct financial incentives from a societal perspective.

pharmaceutical manufacturers from investing in this therapeutic area (Projan and Shlaes 2004). However, others contend that many antibiotics approved for use have not been evaluated adequately. Therefore, showing noninferiority by some specific margin against an intervention that may not be better than a placebo is no indicator of effectiveness at best, and at worst could be worse than a placebo (Powers, Cooper et al. 2005). This report does not address the question of appropriate standards for new antibiotics directly except to point out that the issue of weighing the benefits of having a new drug against safety concerns is not unique to antibiotics.[5]

However, FDA does have a role in ensuring patient safety by making new antibiotics available for pathogens that are not treatable using existing drugs. In this role, an objective of FDA's Critical Path Initiative is to ensure faster approval and reverse the declining number of drug approvals each year.[6] Although it certainly makes sense for FDA to do what it can within its protocols to speed up the rate at which antibiotics move through the approval process and lower development costs for pharmaceutical manufacturers, the faster rate of

---

4 In truth, there is no lack of targets; the problem lies in the ability to create a drug that can attack those targets without being toxic to the patient.

5 Safety concerns have arisen after a new antibiotic has been approved, as was the case with Ketek, a macrolide introduced by Sanofi-Aventis in 2004. Nevertheless, it is important to ensure that regulations intended to prevent unsafe drugs do not delay new antibiotics in the pipeline. Delays can have significant costs in discouraging manufacturers from investing in this area.

6 http://www.fda.gov/oc/initiatives/criticalpath/whitepaper.pdf.

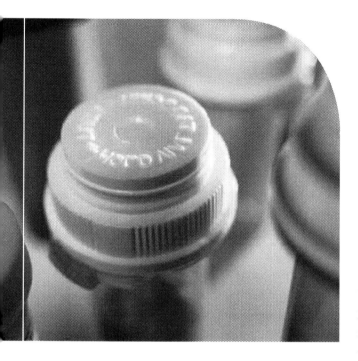

Infectious Diseases Society of America, called for statutory incentives to promote the development of new antibiotics, including tax credits for research and development, wildcard patents that could be used to extend patent life on other "blockbuster" drugs made by the company, lowered cost of clinical trials through FDA flexibility on the evidence necessary to demonstrate safety and efficacy, and liability protections to lower pharmaceutical industry risk, among other measures. However, these incentives did not require any industry commitment to ensure that the new antibiotics would not be overused or marketed for uses that might hasten the emergence of resistance. Nor did they require that the new antibiotics come from new classes rather than from the current 16 classes of compounds. The commons problem that exists when several companies are making related antibiotics having the same genetic basis for resistance was not addressed by this proposed legislation.

An alternative is to tie benefits to pharmaceutical firms to the level of effectiveness of their products. Such measures would give the industry incentive to care more about drug resistance. Providing incentives for new drugs without requiring investments in ensuring appropriate antibiotic use is likely to result in a repeat of the current situation in a decade or two, and moreover, it is unlikely that new drug development can ever keep pace with the rate at which bacteria develop resistance to new drugs. However, the greater the restrictions on new antibiotics, the larger the incentives needed to keep the pharmaceutical industry involved in the pursuit of new antibiotics.

approval could come at the cost of patient safety. Industry incentives to develop new antibiotics are enhanced by faster approval (by reducing the safety and efficacy requirements) or more attractive financial incentives or both. Faster approvals may be less desirable than direct financial incentives from a societal perspective.[7]

Providing economic incentives to encourage firms' research and development on antibiotics is outside the mandate of any federal agency and has to be separately authorized by Congress. The Bioshield II bill[8] cosponsored by Senators Joseph Lieberman and Orrin Hatch, which received strong support from the medical profession, the American Association of Tropical Medicine and Hygiene, and the

Recent legislation by Congress created the Biomedical Advanced Research and Development Agency (BARDA) to act as the "single point of authority" to promote advanced research and development of drugs and vaccines in response to bioterrorism and natural disease outbreaks. The legislation has the potential to encourage new research into antibiotics by shielding drug manufacturers from liability lawsuits if a

---

7    Speeding up approval by FDA without investing more resources in the approval process could compromise patient safety. The hurdle is the massive amount of information that agency staff must absorb about a drug before a reasonably informed determination can be made about its usefulness and safety.

8    http://www.govtrack.us/congress/bill.xpd?bill=s109-975.

> EPA regulations regarding *Bt* are the first from any U.S. agency that treat pest susceptibility as a public good.

drug used to counteract bioterrorism or epidemics caused death or injury. The agency could also potentially fund new drug development directly—with billions of dollars, at a scale similar to the Defense Advanced Research Projects Agency—if the problem of resistance were a national security issue. However, as with Bioshield II (upon which the new bill drew heavily), fundamental problems associated with the common property nature of antibiotic effectiveness and the need to develop new classes of antibiotics are not addressed.[9]

■
_____

## A possible model: EPA and pest resistance to *Bt*

The Environmental Protection Agency (EPA) offers the only example of a federal agency that has regulated for effectiveness of a biological control agent by acting preemptively to prevent the emergence of pest resistance to transgenic crops. The Federal Insecticide, Fungicide, and Rodenticide Act gives EPA authority to amend or revoke existing registrations of pesticides in the event of "unreasonable adverse effects." The law also permits EPA to impose new measures as new information becomes available. EPA has used this law in recent years to regulate for pest resistance to *Bacillus thuringiensis,* or *Bt*. A gene from this bacterium codes for the

production of a protein highly toxic to many insect pests and has been inserted in cotton, tobacco, corn, and soybean varieties. Unlike chemical pesticides, which may be blown away or washed off or lose effectiveness after being sprayed on crops, the pesticide is always present in these *Bt* varieties.

Recognizing the societal value of *Bt* effectiveness, EPA has required manufacturers of *Bt* crops to have insect resistance plans that include a requirement that growers plant an area of non-*Bt* corn or cotton to provide a refuge for susceptible pests[10] (EPA 1998; EPA 2001; Berwald, Matten et al. 2006). Planting a refuge is expected to dilute resistance by allowing mating between pests that may be highly resistant to *Bt* with those that are susceptible. In addition, EPA has required that the seed companies educate growers, have a compliance assurance program and an annual resistance monitoring program, and develop a remedial plan in case resistance is identified (EPA 2001). This is the first instance in which refuge areas have been required by regulation in the United States (Livingston, Carlson et al. 2000).

EPA's resistance management plan has been found to be effective in delaying the emergence of resistance to *Bt* crops and thus far appears successful (Tabashnik, Dennehy et al. 2005). It is interesting that EPA regulations regarding *Bt* are the first from any U.S. agency that treat pest susceptibility as a public good (Livingston et al. 2000), even though resistance issues arose with more traditional pesticides as well.[11] To date,

_____

9   Critics of the legislation have reservations about its provisions to shield the new agency from public Freedom of Information Act requests and exempt it from longstanding and widely applicable laws on open records and public meetings.

10   The refuge requirement for *Bt* cotton has been in place since 1995, and for *Bt* corn since 1998.

11   It is interesting that transgenics triggered policy action but traditional pesticides did not. In both cases, an externality is present: any farmer applying a pesticide is helping to create a resistant pest population that can affect other farmers. The Pesticide Program Dialogue committee in 1996 recommended to EPA that protection of the susceptibility of *Bt* was in the "public good." In response to a lawsuit filed by Greenpeace in 1998, EPA recognized the higher selection intensity posed by transgenic *Bt* plants (since unlike conventional pesticides, a plant-incorporated protectant is always in the environment) and originally was concerned about the protection of microbial pesticides used in organic agriculture. The agency later expanded its concern for all *Bt* pesticides (plant-

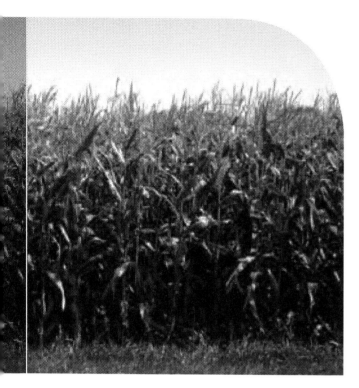

exercised this type of power and has not indicated a willingness to withdraw a drug approval because of emerging resistance to it.[12]

## The nature of a regulatory solution

The basic framework for government action on antibiotics is clearly spelled out in the Antimicrobial Resistance Action Plan formulated by ITFAR.[13] The plan offers steps to changing incentives for both appropriate prescribing and better use of diagnostics to reduce the need for antibiotics. It specifically calls for actions to "identify economic and other barriers in the health care system (e.g., reimbursement policies by third-party payers, managed care practices, cost considerations, empiric treatment recommendations, etc.) to diagnostic testing that promotes appropriate use of antimicrobials" and "develop recommendations that remove disincentives or promote incentives to such testing." It also recognizes that "manufacturers are concerned that appropriate use policies may limit sales and profits" and calls for ways to "identify financial and/or other incentives or investments to promote the development and/or appropriate use of priority antimicrobial resistance products, such as novel compounds and approaches, for human and veterinary medicine for which market incentives are inadequate." Finally, it calls for a consideration of government's role in new drug discovery, especially where market incentives are limited.

Although based on a sound plan, current government response to the problem of antibiotic resistance has been hampered by important constraints. First, no single agency

there have been no major challenges to EPA's authority to regulate for pest resistance to *Bt*. This might indicate that in the interests of society, FDA could similarly regulate use of antibiotics or the conditions under which they are used.

In theory, FDA has sufficient power under current law to regulate for drug resistance in the interests of patient safety as proactively as EPA has regulated the planting of *Bt* crops. Current law permits FDA to grant conditional registrations that can be periodically evaluated to ensure that the registrant is meeting FDA's requirements for ensuring patient safety by minimizing the likelihood of resistance. However, FDA has not

---

incorporated protectants and microbial pesticides). The agency also recognized that *Bt* crops had the potential to displace higher-risk conventional chemical pesticides, and that there was strong public interest to maintain the environmental benefits of lower conventional pesticide use through effective management of *Bt* resistance.

12  The real reason may be a deep cultural difference between medical practice and agriculture. Looking over the shoulders of farmers to ensure that they undertake specific actions that are in the public interest, even if these involve a risk to the farmer's crop, is generally considered acceptable, whereas regulating a doctor's decisions on how to treat an individual patient (even if these actions involve risks to health of others) is not.

13  http://www.cdc.gov/drugresistance/actionplan/.

is charged with responsibility for antibiotic effectiveness. Although the ITFAR plan calls on CDC, FDA, and NIH to coordinate their activities, the agencies' representatives on ITFAR still have to make the case for doing something about antibiotics within their own organizations. Many actions, such as spending more on antibiotic resistance surveillance or basic science to support discovery of new antibiotics, compete with other priorities for staff time, funding, and attention. In other words, just the mandate to CDC, FDA, and NIH to take action to manage drug resistance does not necessarily give them incentive to make large changes and deviate from current structures. A review of ITFAR's goals and achievements over its five years of activity shows that many of the more easily attainable goals have already been reached, but the more difficult steps will require far more commitment and resources. For instance, creating a separate department within FDA to deal with antibiotics may require congressional authorization.

It may be illustrative to look at a model of action on federal management of fisheries. The Magnuson-Stevens Fishery Conservation and Management Act of 1976 declared Congress's interests in "the fish off the coasts of the United States ... [that] constitute valuable and renewable natural resources." The act, which recognizes the economic and food-related importance of fish to the country, called for measures to protect the nation's fisheries and fish habitats through investments in fisheries development, data monitoring systems, fisheries management plans to "achieve and maintain, on a continuing basis, the optimum yield from each fishery," and federal permits, licenses, and other methods.[14] The Magnuson-Stevens Act is by no means a model for managing all resources, and this discussion is meant only to draw attention to the need for comprehensive

legislation to consider antibiotics as a valuable national resource.[15] Moreover, it may be helpful to learn from both the successes and the failures of this earlier effort to manage a common property resource.

Comprehensive legislation to protect antibiotic effectiveness at the federal level would have three important advantages. First, it would recognize a vital national interest in the effectiveness of antibiotics that would signal to federal agencies the legislature's recognition of the importance of this problem. This is crucial because a mandate may not give the agencies sufficient reason to act (although the *Bt* example is one where that did happen); separate mechanisms

---

15 Although several revisions to the act have improved its performance, and the history of U.S. national fisheries is not a success by any standards, it is likely that the situation would have been substantially worse in the absence of the Magnuson-Stevens Act.

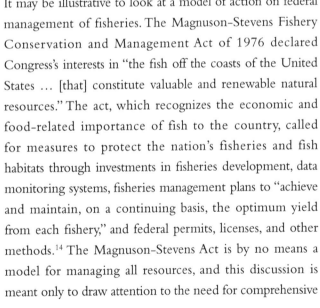

---

14 The Magnuson-Stevens Act was originally motivated by resentment over the presence of foreign fishing fleets off the U.S. coast as much as by concern over depleted fish stocks.

may be necessary. For example, the Magnuson-Stevens Act requires fisheries managers to identify and mitigate adverse impacts of fishing activity on essential fish habitat. Similarly, FDA could identify and mitigate actions that have an adverse impact on drug effectiveness. FDA's 2000 ban on selling fluoroquinolones for poultry can be seen as a precedent (Box 5.1), but this action fell well within FDA's role in protecting patient safety. In a hypothetical situation where the widespread use of one fluoroquinolone in human medicine is responsible for an increased likelihood of resistance to the entire class of quinolones, FDA's willingness to act is less clear.

Second, legislation specifically addressing the problem of antibiotic resistance could provide funding for programs to help conserve the effectiveness of existing drugs and support investments in new drugs. Work to prolong drug effectiveness must compete with other public health and biomedical priorities, and a separate line of funding that would pay for surveillance of resistance in hospitals and communities would help both public health officials and pharmaceutical firms in determining the need for new drugs. CDC, NIH, and FDA need funding for proactive measures to manage drug effectiveness as well.

Third, legislation would tie together actions to manage antibiotic effectiveness and those to improve the supply of new antibiotics, recognizing the impact of demand-side measures on supplier incentives and vice versa. Despite the advantages of the current regulatory structure, which links to other public health functions (such as CDC's role in responding to disease outbreaks), a coordinating body that bridges the mandates of existing institutions and reports directly to the secretary of Health and Human Services may be necessary.

## CONCLUSIONS

The antibiotic resistance problem involves a common property resource—antibiotic effectiveness—that is likely being overexploited. Since resistant strains generated in one state can affect other states, federal action is appropriate. Federal agencies, most notably CDC and FDA, may have a mandate sufficient to undertake many of the actions needed to respond to the threat of resistance. The problem, however, is that they have weak incentives to do so and other priorities. Moreover, some remedies—such as giving pharmaceutical companies incentives to invest in new classes of antibiotics and relaxing antitrust or expanding patent scope to give them incentives to care about resistance—exceed the agencies' current mandates and would require action by Congress.

This report offers many specific policy ideas (Chapters 3, 4, 6, and 7). Pulling them all together into a coordinated response at the federal level may require new, comprehensive legislation specifically addressing antibiotic resistance. The problem is conserving a national resource, and piecemeal remedies, such as bills that create incentives for pharmaceutical companies (like the proposed Bioshield II legislation) or reduce inappropriate antibiotic use in livestock, may not be adequate.

# References

Berwald, D., S. Matten, et al. (2006). Economic Analysis and Regulating Pesticide Biotechnology at the U.S. Environmental Protection Agency. *Regulating Agricultural Biotechnology: Economics and Policy.* Just, R. E., J. M. Alston, et al. (eds.). Vol. 30 of *Natural Resources Management and Policy.* New York, NY: Springer US, 1-15.

EPA. (1998). The Environment Protection Agency's White Paper on *Bt* Plant-Pesticide Resistance Management. Washington, DC: EPA. U.S. Environmental Protection Agency.

————. (2001). "Biopesticides Registration Action Document: *Bacillus thuringiensis* Plant-Incorporated Protectants." http://www.epa.gov/pesticides/biopesticides/pips/Bt_brad.htm (accessed May 31, 1976).

Livingston, M. J., G. A. Carlson, et al. (2000). Bt *Cotton Refuge Policy.* Presented at the American Agricultural Economics Association Meetings, Tampa Bay, FL.

Powers, J. H., C. K. Cooper, et al. (2005). "Sample Size and the Ethics of Non-Inferiority Trials." *Lancet* 366(9479): 24-5.

Projan, S. J. and D. M. Shlaes. (2004). "Antibacterial Drug Discovery: Is It All Downhill From Here?" *Clinical Microbiology and Infection* 10(Suppl 4): 18-22.

Spellberg, B., J. H. Powers, et al. (2004). "Trends in Antimicrobial Drug Development: Implications for the Future." *Clinical Infectious Diseases* 38(9): 1279-86.

Tabashnik, B. E., T. J. Dennehy, et al. (2005). "Delayed Resistance to Transgenic Cotton in Pink Bollworm." *Proceedings of the National Academy of Sciences of the United States of America* 102(43): 15389-93.

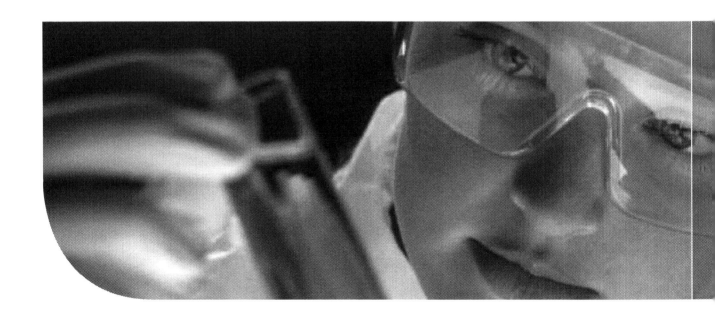

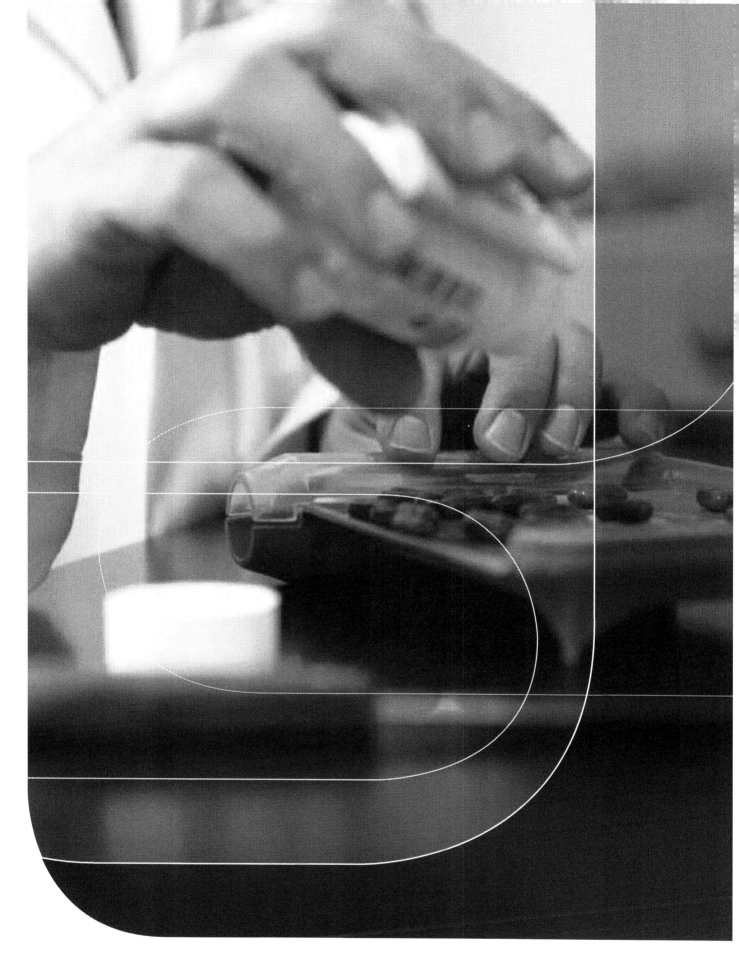

# The role of **health insurance**

*Anup Malani*

This chapter examines the role that health insurance, especially the government programs Medicare and Medicaid, might play in controlling antibiotic resistance. The central problem with antibiotic use by one patient is that it may have a negative externality—the spread of a resistant infection to other patients. If, however, those patients are part of the same health insurance pool, the health insurance company will "internalize" those effects and therefore have an incentive to promote the socially optimal level of antibiotic use.

The two federal government health insurance programs are in a unique position to manage the externalities from antibiotic use. Medicare is the nation's largest unified insurer. Moreover, because Medicare and Medicaid together are such large purchasers of medical care, they have the bargaining power to effect significant changes in the conduct of doctors and hospitals. At the very least, because they have high visibility, they can take a leadership role in highlighting the importance of ensuring the socially optimal use of antibiotics.

It is important, however, to note the difficulties with employing Medicare and Medicaid as instruments to limit the growth of resistance. One is that government agencies likely do not respond as well as private firms to incentives to control costs, in this case from resistance. Another is that Medicare, which is better able to coordinate a response to resistance than Medicaid, does not cover long-term care facilities, which are a significant source of antibiotic use and resistance.

This chapter is organized into seven sections. The first explains why health insurance companies might find it in their interest to control the externalities from antibiotic use. The second presents some limitations on the scope of health insurance companies and thus on their ability to control antibiotic-related externalities. The third section explains

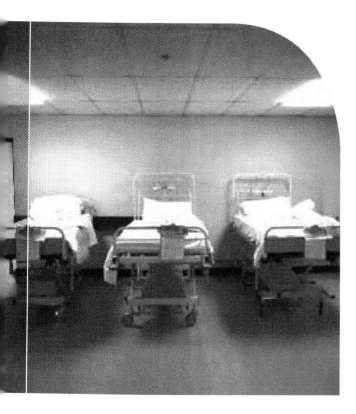

why, among health plans, Medicare and Medicaid might be uniquely positioned to control resistance externalities from antibiotic use. The next section reviews existing quality control programs that could serve as models for programs to control antibiotic resistance, and the following section explores ideas for new programs specifically targeting the problem. The penultimate section reviews the limitations of Medicare and Medicaid. The conclusion explores alternative mechanisms to internalize the externalities from antibiotic use.

■

## Background

The public policy concern with antibiotics is driven by the externalities from their use, one positive and one negative. To simplify, the positive externality is that patient A's use of an antibiotic against a contagious bacterial infection prevents the spread of that infection to patient B. The negative externality is that patient A's use (or misuse) of an antibiotic may make the bacteria in her body resistant to the antibiotic, and these resistant bacteria may spread to patient B. Because the bacteria are now resistant to the antibiotic that A used, B cannot use that antibiotic to control his infection.

A standard solution to an externality is to get the source of the externality to "internalize" the external benefits or costs she imposes on others. If the source bears all the external effects of her decision, she will behave in a manner that is consistent with social welfare—that is, the good of the community and not just herself. To demonstrate how this might work, consider the classic example of the rancher who is neighbors with a farmer (Coase 1960). The externality is that the rancher's cattle occasionally wander onto the farmer's land and trample his crops. There are many ways to get the ranching business to internalize its externality on the farm. For example, the farmer could buy the rancher's business or sue the rancher in tort for damage to his crops. If the value of the lost crops is greater than the value of additional grazing opportunities for cattle, then the grazing will voluntarily cease.[1]

The problem with applying this solution to the antibiotic problem is that it is not immediately obvious how to get one patient to internalize the externalities of her antibiotic use on the other patient. Moreover, allowing one patient to sue another is complicated by two problems.[2] First, litigation

---

1   Another solution is to regulate the behavior or environment of the source to control her externalities. In the rancher and farmer example, the alternative to internalization is mandatory government regulation that, for instance, requires ranchers to fence their property or limits cattle populations. In the antibiotic context, the government could tax antibiotic use or require better sanitation.

2   People can and do sue hospitals for hospital-acquired infections. In one view, this strategy holds hospitals vicariously liable for externalities that emanate from patients. In another view, hospitals (or their agents, nurses, and nonindependent contractor doctors) are liable for infections because they are delegated the task of treatment by patients. In either case, the purpose of liability is to encourage hospitals to control infections and to manage antibiotic use. Some obvious limitations of the strategy are that

is traditionally used to manage only negative externalities—damages as opposed to windfalls. Second, whereas it is easy to determine whether the rancher's cattle harmed his neighbor's crops, it is hard to determine which other patient's antibiotic use is responsible for a victim's resistant bacterial infection.

Nevertheless, there may be an indirect way to ensure that antibiotic externalities are internalized. Most patients do not directly pay for their medical care. Rather, their health insurance plan pays for the cost of treatment. In most cases, patients pay an annual premium (in monthly installments) and the health insurance company pays for each treatment as required. If a patient acquires a bacterial infection, whether resistant or otherwise, the health insurance company bears the marginal cost of treatment of that infection. Moreover, if patients A and B purchase health insurance plans from the same company and thus are in the same insurance pool, then that company internalizes the health expense behavior of both patients. If A uses an antibiotic, the company pays for it. If this prevents a nonresistant bacterial infection in B, the company avoids paying for treatment of that infection. If it causes a resistant infection in B, then the company pays for the cost of his treatment. Therefore, the company has an incentive to subsidize consumption of an antibiotic when it has a positive externality because it lowers the costs of treating other patients. Likewise, it has an incentive to limit consumption of an antibiotic when it has a negative externality because that would increase the cost of treating other patients.[3] In short, health insurance may be a vehicle for internalizing the externalities from antibiotic use.

## Limitations to using health insurance

That said, there are several limitations on the use of health insurance to manage the external effects of antibiotic use. First, some costs of bacterial infections—days off work, pain and suffering—may not be insured.[4] The magnitude of this omission may be quite large. For evidence we can look to medical malpractice cases. Compensatory damages from malpractice are divided into two categories, economic and noneconomic. Economic damages include cost of medical care and loss of wages; noneconomic damages include pain and suffering. A 2004 RAND study of medical malpractice jury verdicts in California found that the average award for noneconomic damages was 72 percent of the average award for economic damages (Pace, Golinelli et al. 2004). This suggests that the nonmedical costs of bacterial infections may be less than 42 percent of the total costs of these infections.[5] Although medical malpractice injuries may not be representative of all injuries and jury verdicts may be somewhat imprecise,[6] the statistics suggest that health insurance companies may not fully internalize the costs of third-party bacterial infections.

The incomplete scope of coverage does not necessarily sink health insurance as a vehicle for regulating externalities. If the noncovered costs of the positive versus negative externalities are roughly proportional to the covered costs

---

it does not address the problem of community-acquired infections or of patients admitted with resistant infections acquired at other hospitals (not the fault of the hospital being sued). Indeed, it is possible that liability exposure may encourage hospitals to avoid patients with a history of resistance. Nevertheless, the possibility of internalizing infection externalities through litigation should be explored. It is, however, outside the scope of this chapter.

3  Of course, insurance companies cannot stop patients from consuming antibiotics that are purchased over the counter.

4  Indeed, the to-the-bone cynic might argue that one cost—mortality—actually encourages the health insurance company to always undertreat in the hopes of reducing costs. This perverse incentive is limited by the Consolidated Omnibus Budget Reconciliation Act of 1985, which allows an employee's surviving spouse to purchase continuation coverage, 29 U.S.C.A. §1163, at virtually the same premium, §§1162(3), 1164, for 18 months, §1162(2).

5  It is possible that the noneconomic damages include not just the nonmedical costs of malpractice, but also, for example, the "outrage" the jury feels towards the defendant's behavior or other "justice"-related concerns. Nevertheless, a nontrivial portion of noneconomic damages also includes nonmedical costs.

6  But see Vidmar (1995).

of these externalities, then heath insurers may still have the proper incentives to balance these externalities. Although the findings of studies that examine the effects of resistant and nonresistant infections vary widely, a recent study by Cosgrove, Qi et al. (2005) is fairly representative. That study found that methicillin-resistant *Staphylococcus aureus* (MRSA) increased the length of hospital stay and hospital charges by similar numbers, 29 and 36 percent, respectively, relative to methicillin-susceptible *S. aureus* (MSSA).[7] Thus there may be a rough balance in relative impact of resistant infections on covered outcomes (hospital charges) and noncovered outcomes (length of stay and thus wages), which are proportional to length of stay. Therefore, the incomplete coverage may not significantly skew the incentives of health insurers to achieve the social optimum.

A second problem with using health insurance to control antibiotic externalities is that no health insurance plan covers all third parties that might be affected by a covered individual's antibiotic use. Therefore, no insurance plan will account for the external effect of a beneficiary's antibiotic use on all third parties. The largest private insurer, UnitedHealth Group, covers about 65 million persons nationwide (WSJ. com 2006). This is, to be sure, a very high number. But no other company comes close to UnitedHealth's market share. Moreover, unlike the externalities from antibiotic use, UnitedHealth's market share is not geographically concentrated. If it were, it could face significant antitrust liability.

A third problem with internalization through health insurance is that most insurance contracts have limited duration.

Therefore, insurers do not have the incentive to account for the externalities suffered by (as opposed to those caused by) an individual that occur after her contract terminates. In general, insurance contracts have a duration of one year. Because most health insurance is provided as an employee benefit, however, the actual length of coverage is the length of employment at a given employer. Moreover, under the Consolidated Omnibus Budget Reconciliation Act (COBRA) of 1985, an employee generally has the right to purchase 18 months of continuation coverage from the same insurance company, 29 U.S.C.A. §1162. Finally, many employees have retiree coverage. According to the U.S. Census Bureau (2006), of the 34.7 million persons over the age of 65 in 2003, 12.2 million had private health insurance related to their employment. Regardless of the length of an individual's health insurance contract, however, and even with COBRA, coverage ends 18 months after retirement unless the individual has retiree coverage through his employer. And it is unheard of for an individual—other than one associated with the military—to have cradle-to-grave insurance coverage from the same company. Therefore, even a covered person's life includes significant periods that are not incorporated into an insurance company's calculus of the net benefit of antibiotic use.

Like the problem of incomplete scope of coverage, neither the nonuniversal nature of coverage nor its incomplete duration renders health insurance useless as a vehicle to internalize the external effects of antibiotic use. At most, the limitations make it a somewhat worse second-best remedy.[8] The loss from incomplete duration and nonuniversal coverage is limited so

---

7  At least for MRSA, the results on mortality are scattered. Along with McHugh and Riley (2004), Cosgrove, Qi et al. (2005) found no effect of resistance on mortality. However, Engemann, Carmeli et al. (2003) found a threefold increase in mortality relative to MSSA for surgical-site MRSA. Finally, Pittet, Tarara et al. (1994) and Pittet and Wenzel (1995) report that patients with a nosocomial bloodstream infection are 35 percent more likely to die.

8  That said, there is an asymmetric risk that current health insurance may contribute to the overuse of antibiotics. The first-order effect of insurance is to reduce the marginal cost of antibiotic use and thus encourage more consumption than may be optimal, given the negative resistance externalities of antibiotic use (see Chapter 2). If the net external effect of antibiotic use is negative, antibiotics should be subject to a Pigovian tax rather than a subsidy, it may be hard for an insurance company to levy such a tax because a patient could simply purchase the antibiotic on her own without telling the insurance company. It would be difficult for insurance companies to enforce contractual limitations on such sales.

> Because of their size, Medicare and Medicaid have greater incentives than private insurance plans to internalize the costs of antibiotic use.

long as either the external benefits or the external costs of antibiotic use are not relatively concentrated in covered life years. For example, if covered life years tend to capture only the positive externalities from antibiotic use—that is, covered lives are mainly at risk from nonresistant infections—then health insurance policies will be biased in favor of excessive use of antibiotics.

■ _____

## The unique potential of Medicare and Medicaid

Given that the incentive of health insurance plans to correctly control externalities from antibiotic use is proportional to coverage, the limitations of current private health insurance plans highlight a potential benefit from a universal health insurance plan, whether run by the government or by a private entity. Since our focus is the problem of drug resistance, the pros and cons of universal health insurance are outside the scope of this discussion. Instead, this chapter focuses on the next best thing: Medicare and Medicaid.

Medicare is primarily a federally run, mandatory old-age and disability insurance program. Medicaid is primarily a state-run welfare program that pays for health care for the poor. Each program has a different structure, and each structure has its own complexities (Box 6.1 and Box 6.2). Although Medicare and Medicaid do not have a significantly broader scope of coverage than private plans, they do have two

advantages for the purpose of creating proper incentives to internalize the external effects of antibiotic use.

First, the duration of coverage under the programs is relatively long. Medicare covers individuals from the time they reach the age of 65 to the day they die, 42 U.S.C.A. §426(a). In addition, Medicare covers the disabled for as long as they are disabled, §426(b), and Medicaid covers certain classes of poor people so long as they are poor. Since many disabilities are permanent and the ailments that afflict Medicaid recipients typically reduce their incomes, coverage for disabled persons and for the poor is typically long-lived. Second, the two programs cover a large number of lives. According to the U.S. Census Bureau (2006), Medicare covered 39.5 million persons, and Medicaid, 35.5 million persons in 2003. Because Medicare and Medicaid beneficiaries tend to be medically more vulnerable, although these programs cover only 26 percent of the U.S. population of 288.3 million in 2003, they paid for 47 percent of the cost of all hospital care and 64 percent of the cost of all nursing home care that year (U.S. Census 2006).[9]

Because of their size, Medicare and Medicaid have greater incentives than private insurance plans to internalize the costs of antibiotic use. In addition, however, their immense buying power gives them a great deal of influence over the behavior of providers even with respect to persons *not* covered by these programs. Medicare and Medicaid can directly require, for example, broad infection control programs as a condition of participation. Such programs would benefit not only Medicare and Medicaid enrollees but also other patients. Institutional providers, such as hospitals, would face the prospect of losing half or more of their revenues unless they complied, even though compliance would increase costs for

_____

9  Medicare did the heavy lifting of hospital care costs (30 percent of all costs) and Medicaid did the heavy lifting of nursing home costs (46 percent). The two programs' share of physicians' costs (27 percent) was roughly in line with their population shares.

BOX 6.1

## MEDICARE

Medicare covers two classes of individuals. One class comprises all individuals above the age of 65. Medicare will cover only expenses not otherwise covered by employment-related health insurance for these individuals. The other class includes all disabled persons who have been eligible for Social Security benefits for at least two years. It also includes all individuals with end-stage renal (kidney) disease after a three-month waiting period.

Medicare has four parts. Part A covers inpatient hospital care, care at rehabilitation hospitals, and care at skilled-nursing facilities. It does not, in general, cover care at nursing homes. The distinction between hospitals, skilled-nursing facilities, and nursing homes is that the first are acute care facilities, the second are intermediate care facilities that "pit stop" between hospitals and nursing homes, and nursing homes are long-term care facilities. Home health services are covered partly by Part A and partly by Part B. The latter primarily covers outpatient care at hospitals, physician care, and certain other specialized services, such as home dialysis. Part C, also called the Medicare Advantage (previously the Medicare+Choice) program, is a series of managed-care, prepaid health plans that not only cover all the benefits in Parts A and B but also may offer additional supplemental benefits, including prescription drug coverage. Part D is the new Medicare drug benefit enacted in 2003. It covers some of the cost of prescription drugs outside the hospital setting. (Drugs prescribed pursuant to inpatient hospital services are covered by Part A.) There is also a class of insurance called MediGap that covers services not otherwise covered by Parts A and B.[1]

Part A coverage is primarily financed by the Medicare payroll taxes that individuals pay throughout their lives. It is automatic for those individuals eligible for Medicare.[2] Part B coverage is not automatic: it is available only to those individuals who enroll and pay a Part B premium that only partly covers the cost of the program. (Medicaid typically picks up the premium for low-income enrollees.) The remainder is financed out of general revenues. Part C is an alternative to Part A and Part B. It is offered by private health insurance companies and available to individuals who opt for it and pay a premium to these companies. The essential tradeoff is that individuals typically pay a lower premium than under Part B and/or get broader coverage than Part A and B, but in return they must accept the treatment constraints of managed care. Finally, Part D is financed by and available to any individual who pays a somewhat complicated scheme of premiums, deductibles, and coinsurance.[3] These fees are discounted for low-income individuals.

---

1  MediGap is a supplemental insurance for which individuals must pay separately. The government's basic role in this market is to standardize the 10 basic insurance plans that private companies may offer. The purpose of government regulation is to simplify the choices available to seniors.

2  One caveat is that if an individual has paid less than 40 quarters of Medicare taxes, then she may be charged a premium for Part A benefits.

3  Monthly premiums are roughly $35, and the deductible is $250. There is a 25 percent coinsurance for the next $2,000 of drug expenses, a 100 percent coinsurance for the next $2,850 of drug expenses (popularly known as the "doughnut hole"), and a 5 percent coinsurance for drug expenses in excess of $5,100 (Kaplan 2005).

Medicare coverage and premiums for all parts but C are ultimately set by the Centers for Medicare and Medicaid Services (CMS), a part of the Department of Health and Human Services. Claims are processed and providers are paid, however, by private contractors, such as Blue Cross and Blue Shield associations. Because CMS handles only high-level (or appealed) coverage issues, many applied coverage decisions are made by these private contractors. Because each contractor covers a particular geographic area, Medicare coverage may not be perfectly uniform across the country.

Institutional health care providers, such as hospitals, certain nursing facilities, and home health agencies, must enter into provider agreements to participate in Medicare. These agreements impose certain conditions. For our purposes the most relevant are that providers be "certified" and that they contract with a private peer-review organization to conduct quality and utilization review. For most facilities, the certification requirement is satisfied by seeking accreditation from the Joint Commission on the Accreditation of Health care Organizations (JCAHO), a private accreditation organization that is governed by members of, for example, the American Medical Association and the American Hospital Association. (The JCAHO accreditation process focuses not on health outcomes so much as whether a facility has the resources to provide quality care.) Doctors and pharmacies are not required to sign contracts with Medicare to participate in the program.

all patients. Few providers could stand up to that pressure.

Medicare and Medicaid can also indirectly affect provider behavior. If Medicare and Medicaid were to require, for example, the use of heterogeneous or shorter duration antibiotic therapies for their enrollees, providers would have two reasons to employ the same therapies for patients not covered by the government. First, it is easier for providers to use the same techniques for all patients rather than modify treatment based on the identity of the patient's insurance company.[10] Second, Medicare and Medicaid can change the standard of care by which doctors are judged in medical malpractice cases. Most state courts hold doctors to standards defined, in part, by custom (Peters 2002). But by changing the behavior of a quarter or more of doctors who treat Medicare and Medicaid patients, these programs can change the custom of care.

◼

## Current quality control programs in Medicare

This section describes the various quality control measures implemented by Medicare that might serve as antecedents for antibiotic control measures.

Three basic sources of authority govern Medicare's quality control programs. The first is the Medicare statute that, in addition to setting some basic conditions that hospitals must meet to participate in Medicare, authorizes the U.S. Department of Health and Human Services (HHS) to "impose additional requirements if they are found necessary in the interest of the health and safety of the individuals who are furnished services in hospitals," 42 U.S.C. §1995x(e); 42 C.F.R. 421.1(1)(a)(i) (2005).[11] Recently, Medicare used this

---

10   This is consistent with research by Heidenreich, McClellan et al. (2002), who found that HMO treatment guidelines influence care of nonenrollees who suffer myocardial infarction.

11   Medicare does not have a direct relationship with doctors, as it does with hospitals. The only relationship is indirect: a doctor who accepts

## MEDICAID

In general, Medicaid covers two categories of people: the categorically needy and the medically needy. The categorically needy are mainly poor pregnant women, poor families with children, and the elderly and disabled who are poor. The medically needy are individuals not eligible for welfare benefits based on income but who are nonetheless impoverished because of medical expenses. The main group of poor persons omitted from Medicaid coverage consists of nonelderly, nondisabled persons without children. Because Medicaid is administered by states, specific eligibility criteria vary. Although federal rules mandate that certain groups be covered, states have the option to cover others. Moreover, under the so-called Section 1115 waiver, eligibility is determined solely by negotiations between a state and the Department of Health and Human Services.

Medicaid covers everything in Medicare Parts A and B and more. For example, it also covers family planning and long-term care at nursing homes. At a state's option, it may also cover prescription drugs. For the elderly, it covers Medicare Part A and Part B premiums, as well as long-term nursing home care that is not included in Medicare. Importantly, roughly 50 percent of nursing home residents are on Medicaid (Furrow et al. 2004).

Unlike Medicare, Medicaid is not an insurance plan. Rather, it is an entitlement, which means it is funded entirely from general government revenue. It does not charge beneficiaries any premium, deductible, or coinsurance. The costs of Medicaid are split between the states and the federal government, which contributes 50 to 83 percent of funds, depending on the per capita income of a state (Furrow et al. 2000). Medicaid is administered by each of the 50 states. Subject to certain federal guidelines, states determine eligibility, benefits, and provider reimbursement, and thus the program varies across the country.

mandate to implement the so-called Quality Assessment and Performance Improvement (QAPI) program, 42 C.F.R. §482.21. This program requires hospitals to track quality indicators, such as health outcomes and medical errors; use the data to identify opportunities for improving the quality of patient care and the causes of medical error; adopt programs designed to act on the data; and hold executives and medical staff accountable for implementation of these programs.

Second, the Medicare statute has a Medical Utilization and Quality Control Program, 42 U.S.C. §1320c-1–c-19. Related to this, the statute requires HHS to contract with peer-review organizations (now called quality improvement organizations, QIOs[12]) to monitor hospitals and other

---

assignment of a beneficiary's claim so as to secure payment directly from Medicare must agree not to bill the patient for any unpaid portion of her bill. This narrow relationship limits the extent to which Medicare can change the behavior of individual physicians.

---

12 A list of QIOs can be found at http://www.medqic.org/dcs/Content Server?pagename=Medqic/MQGeneralPage/GeneralPageTemplate&name=QIO%20Listings.

institutional providers to ensure that their services meet coverage criteria and promote effective, efficient, economical, and quality health care, §1395y(g). Medicare has contracted with 53 such organizations to review the health care provided to enrollees in all states and territories. If a QIO finds that a service does not meet the utilization or quality standards, it can retrospectively deny Medicare payment for that service to the provider, §1320c-3(a)(2). If a provider is found to have engaged in flagrant or repeated violations of quality standards, a QIO may institute proceedings to fine the provider or deny it the right to participate in Medicare, §1320c-5(b).

Third, the Centers for Medicare and Medicaid Services (CMS), a part of the Department of Health and Human Services, has the authority to initiate demonstration programs and studies to improve Medicare payment methodologies and operation, §1395ll. In addition, HHS has authority to offer "incentives to improve safety of care provided to beneficiaries" on a demonstration basis, §1395cc-3.[13] One project initiated under CMS authority is the Premier Hospital Quality Incentive Demonstration. This project provides financial rewards to certain nonprofit hospitals that demonstrate high-quality performance in areas such as treatment for heart attacks, pneumonia, and hip and knee replacements (CMS 2006a). Participating hospitals in the top (second) decile of performance receive a 2 percent (1 percent) bonus on their Medicare payments for measured conditions. Another project is the National Health Information Infrastructure (NHII), a voluntary program; it establishes standards for the sharing and analysis of data on patients and their treatments and outcomes to facilitate more effective clinical decisionmaking and control of diseases that threaten public health (HHS 2006). A third project—similar to QAPI but targeting physicians rather than hospitals and not involving any penalties or

> HHS has authority to offer "incentives to improve safety of care provided to beneficiaries" on a demonstration basis.

rewards—is the Physician Voluntary Reporting Program. This program invites physicians to report certain designated quality-related data from their own practices. For example, physicians are asked to report their timing for administration of antibiotics to patients hospitalized for pneumonia and the frequency with which they give antibiotic prophylaxis to surgical patients (CMS 2005).

Medicare will likely have to rely on one or more of these three powers—its authority to set conditions for participation, contract with peer-review organizations or QIOs, and initiate demonstration projects—to implement a program to control antibiotic use. The difference among them lies in the carrots and sticks they employ to achieve their aims. The penalty for failing to meet the conditions of participation is loss of all sales to the government—a rather blunt instrument. The penalty for noncompliance with QIO standards is retrospective denials of payment—a more narrow and targeted instrument. Finally, the demonstration authority employs bonus payments and subsidies rather than penalties to ensure cooperation. It is more powerful in the context of hospitals whose resources are already stretched to the limit. Because Medicare can allow only limited demonstrations, however, full implementation will typically require additional legislation to provide authority to mandate participation by all providers.

To set up a demonstration antibiotic control program or expand a demonstration to all of Medicare (via legislation), one needs

---

13 This power is called the §646 demonstration authority. Because approval of a §646 demonstration involves a lengthy and complex process, it is preferable to act under CMS's more general demonstration authority (Sage forthcoming).

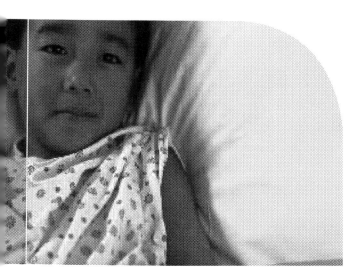

medical residents using a mix of fixed fees and reasonable costs. Specifically, subsidies are based on the number of residents a hospital trains, a hospital's cost of training a resident, the fraction of a hospital's patients who are Medicare enrollees, and the total amount of DRG compensation the hospital received (Bajaj 1999).

---

## What Medicare and Medicaid can do

Medicare and, to a lesser extent, Medicaid can do three things to promote more efficient management of antibiotic use. First, these programs can track bacterial infections, resistance, and antibiotic use among members. Because these programs cover more than 75 million patients, most of whom are poor or elderly and at high risk for resistant infections, they are well positioned to serve as an advance warning system. Second, with their immense purchasing power, they can promote best practices for containing resistance, such as better infection control and extending the life of existing antibiotics. Third, because Medicare is somewhat centrally managed, it can coordinate and serve as a laboratory in which to experiment with different methods for optimizing antibiotic use.

### :: TRACKING ANTIBIOTICS-RELATED OUTCOMES

Medicare already has the best national database for tracking ailments and medical expenditures, the so-called MEDPAR File and Physician/Supplier Procedure Summary Master File, which contains Part A and Part B claims. Because Medicare tracks ailments but not treatment, however, it does not currently permit tracking of antibiotic usage. Medicare Part D will not fully address this gap because it covers only drug prescriptions in the community setting. It therefore misses in-hospital drug use. Moreover, because Medicare tracks only ailments defined by diagnosis-related groups for hospitals and common procedure terminology (CPTs) for physicians, and these codes neither identify nosocomial infections nor distinguish susceptible from resistant bacterial

a method for paying providers for their cooperation. There are currently three models for paying Medicare institutional providers; each is illustrated in Medicare compensation of hospitals.[14] Medicare primarily pays hospitals on a prospective-pay system that offers a fixed fee per ailment, regardless of the actual cost of treatment. Specifically, ailments, such as heart attacks or ulcers, are categorized into diagnosis-related groups (DRGs), and each DRG is associated with a fixed level of compensation. Medicare also compensates hospitals for reasonable capital costs and regional variations in labor costs by adjusting their total DRG payments upon filing proof of these costs.[15] Finally, Medicare subsidizes hospital training of

---

14 Institutions are compensated for longer-term care on a reasonable (or "necessary") cost basis, not the prospective pay system. Some physician services are reimbursed according to reasonable charges by the provider or customary charges by physicians. Other services are reimbursed on the basis of a fee schedule devised by CMS. Just as hospital procedures must be categorized into diagnosis-related groups (DRGs), physician services must be categorized into common procedure terminology (CPT) codes to be reimbursed. Medicare covers 80 percent of charges or fees; the enrollee is responsible for the remaining 20 percent.

15 Medicare monitors capital and labor costs by requiring hospitals to file detailed income statements and balance sheets through the Health care Cost Report Information System. These accounts are periodically audited by Medicare to ensure their accuracy.

infections, the program does not currently facilitate tracking of resistant infections.

A natural solution is to create DRG and CPT codes that correspond to nosocomial and resistant bacterial infections, as well as to the use of antibiotics. The Physician Voluntary Reporting Program demonstration is designed to test this approach. It requires participating doctors to report not just CPT codes when filing claims, but also a "G-code," which will track, for example, whether a patient was eligible for and received an antibiotic prophylaxis prior to surgery (CMS 2006b). However, one must be careful when making the Medicare fee structure sensitive to antibiotic-related codes lest one generate moral hazard. For example, if nosocomial (hospital-acquired) infections are separately compensated, hospitals may be less vigilant against these infections because they can generate additional payments from Medicare. Conversely, if nosocomial (hospital-acquired) infections are penalized, then hospitals may be discouraged from diagnosing or reporting them.

Several alternative strategies are less likely to be complicated by moral hazard in treatment. For example, Medicare could add nosocomial and resistant infections, as well as antibiotic prescriptions, to QAPI. The problem is that the penalty for failing to comply, disallowing participation in Medicare, is rather blunt. Another approach would be to require contracting QIOs to retrospectively deny payments for existing DRGs if they detect, during utilization review, that a provider has, for example, employed second-line or reserved antibiotics without performing a blood culture or without reporting antibiotic use directly to a registry, such as the National Nosocomial Infection Surveillance system run by the Centers for Disease Control and Prevention. This solution is both feasible and reasonable. Its only limitation is the frequency with which QIOs conduct utilization review. If the frequency is low, the incentive will be weak because the penalty for failing utilization review is effectively capped

at the fee for those patient admissions that are reviewed by the QIO. A third option is to extend the National Health Information Infrastructure to cover antibiotics-related outcomes. The main advantage of NHII is that it would ensure that reports across hospitals are uniform and comparable. The disadvantage of NHII is that it is voluntary. As such, it is not much of an improvement over the National Nosocomial Infection Surveillance program, which is also voluntary and has a very low response rate on antibiotics-related questions.[16] For NHII to make a difference, it must either be coupled with greater financial incentives or be made mandatory.

## :: PROMOTING BEST PRACTICES

A second task for Medicare is to promote best practices for antibiotic use. One category of best practice includes activities that resemble fixed costs, such as formulary controls to centrally manage antibiotic use. These controls can limit use or help cycle antibiotics over patients within a hospital to reduce the probability that a resistant infection cannot be treated by any antibiotic (Laxminarayan 2001).[17] The category also includes infection control activities, such as active surveillance of all incoming patients, regulations to encourage hand washing by hospital staff, and the convenient placement of sinks.

The second category includes patient-specific activities that are akin to incremental or marginal costs, such as blood cultures for sore throats, coughs, and the like to ensure

---

16    Phone conversation with Daniel Pollack, Health care Outcomes Branch Chief, Division of Health care Quality Promotion, National Center for Infectious Diseases, CDC, January 27, 2006.

17    Such controls are especially valuable for ear infections, sinusitis, and bronchitis—situations where blood cultures cannot usually be obtained. Lieberman and Wootan. (1998) suggest that use guidelines be developed by HHS directly rather than by hospitals. Although this would economize on the costs of developing guidelines and ensure uniformity across hospitals, such regulations may be harder for Medicare to police. Medicare could employ QIOs to punish violations, but utilization review is costly and therefore infrequent.

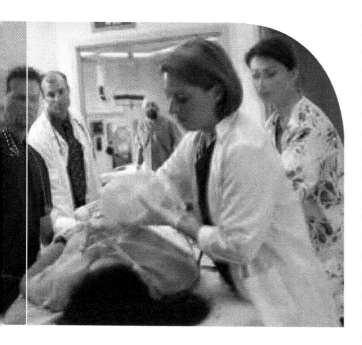

Practices in the incremental cost category are best encouraged either by utilization review (a stick) to ensure compliance with HHS practice guidelines requiring, for example, more blood cultures, or by creating independently billable DRGs (a carrot) that explicitly require and reward use of shorter duration or combination therapies if they are effective. It is particularly important for Medicaid to encourage practices in this category by raising compensation for blood cultures and more effective methods of using antibiotics. Whereas Medicare can encourage hospitals to incur fixed costs that also benefit Medicare patients, it cannot do the same for incremental costs with respect to low-income, nonelderly patients. The problem is that Medicaid reimbursement rates are very low and therefore have little power to encourage better practices. The remedy is to move to reimbursement rates that reflect market prices but that may not be financially (or politically) feasible.

The rationale for this matching is that it would be difficult to encourage fixed costs with utilization review or DRGs alone. It is hard to tell from utilization review of a small number of medical cases whether a hospital has failed to adopt formulary controls or has simply failed to enforce those controls in the sampled cases. Moreover, because the costs of these programs depend not so much on the number of Medicare patients or how sick these patients are as on simply the size of the facility, it would be hard to find a formula for DRG-based fees that would neither under- nor overcompensate. Conversely, it would not make sense to employ the conditions of participation power to encourage more blood cultures. For one thing, Medicare does not have an extensive monitoring system to ensure ongoing compliance with conditions of participation. For another problem, it would not be credible for Medicare to deny a hospital all participation in Medicare for failing to comply with rules for one specific type of ailment.

An alternative to creating incentives for specific best practices is to reward certain outcomes and let providers choose how to

that antibiotics are used only when necessary, and shorter duration therapies (if they are effective) to reduce the probability that bacteria will evolve resistance to antibiotics. It also includes vaccinating patients at risk for pneumococcal infections to reduce the demand for antibiotics to control them. Finally, the category includes judicious use of certain catheters (indwelling bladder catheters and central venous catheters) that are major risk factors for resistant infections (Stosor, Peterson et al. 1998; McHugh and Riley 2004).

The purpose of dividing practices into fixed and incremental cost categories is to match practices with incentives and methods of financing that are best suited to promote them. Practices in the fixed cost category are best encouraged by employing Medicare's "conditions of participation" power (a stick) or reimbursing hospitals for capital costs (a carrot). The former would deny a provider the privilege of participating in Medicare if, for example, it failed to develop formulary controls. The latter could finance the installment of sinks and the use of rapid diagnostic tests for active surveillance.

achieve them. For example, Medicare could require reporting of bacterial infections, their susceptibility to antibiotics, and whether they are community-acquired or nosocomial. If an institution falls below acceptable levels or fails to demonstrate improvement from baseline in these statistics, Medicare could make adjustments in total DRG compensation, much as Medicare does to account for capital and labor costs. The advantage of this approach is that it encourages hospitals to choose the best combination of methods to control susceptible and resistant infections. If hospitals have better information than CMS about local conditions and if local conditions play an important role in controlling infections, then this strategy may be more effective than a process-based incentive system.

A disadvantage, however, is that hospitals and physicians might game the outcome-based scheme by trying to avoid patients with bacterial infections (Dranove, Kessler et al. 2003) or by refusing to monitor and report thoroughly the rate of nosocomial infections. Moreover, because infectious diseases are not confined to institutions, hospitals and nursing homes may have externalities on one another (Smith, Levin et al. 2005). An incentive scheme that pays or punishes for performance only at the target provider will not be able to account for these externalities. Even if the scheme did account for outcomes at other providers—for example, by examining claims from all the Medicare providers that treated a Medicare enrollee who was diagnosed with a resistant infection—it may be difficult to assign blame and thus payoffs among providers. Medicare does not currently have a record of each patient's antibiotic usage. Even if it did, other problems would arise. If providers do not also have a patient's complete history of antibiotics usage, it would be difficult to determine whether antibiotic use is net beneficial; a Medicare incentive could not change that. Finally, if a patient does not have a history of antibiotic usage, she may have caught the infection from another patient. If this happened in the community, Medicare could not assign responsibility to any particular provider. One solution is for Medicare to

simply give bonuses or impose penalties for all providers in a geographic vicinity based on prevalence of infection in that area. Unless the bonuses or penalties were very high, however, such a scheme would give inadequate incentives to control antibiotic use because the cost of poor practices would then be borne by others.

## :: BEING A LABORATORY FOR INNOVATION

A third role for Medicare is experimentation with different methods of infection and resistance control. Because Medicare is centrally managed, it could ask similarly situated hospitals to try different control strategies, pool the information on their results, and determine which methods are superior. For example, Medicare could request that providers in different areas try different formulary management strategies to determine which strategy is most likely to reduce the risk that resistance develops. It could compare areas that employ strategies that require rotation of antibiotics with areas that do not to determine whether heterogeneous use of antibiotics delays emergence of resistance.[18] Such experimentation can be authorized using HHS's existing demonstration power. The main challenge for such experiments is that prior demonstrations have been voluntary, and voluntary participation introduces selection bias into inferences from experiments. The difficulty is not that participating providers cannot be randomized to different "treatments," but that the providers that volunteer for a demonstration may not be representative of nonparticipants. As such, the results of experiments may have limited external validity. One solution is to ensure that the payment for participation is sufficiently large that all providers want to participate—a costly proposition. The alternative is to make the demonstration mandatory. It is unclear, however, whether HHS has the

---

18 This sort of experimentation need not be confined to questions concerning antibiotic resistance. And its use to promote resistance control can certainly be a model for experimentation relevant to other quality control issues.

> **Neither Medicare nor Medicaid has thus far made a serious attempt to control the externalities of antibiotic use.**

power to require participation in a demonstration, let alone a demonstration that involves experimentation with, for example, different therapies.

## Limitations to using Medicare and Medicaid

Although Medicare and Medicaid, because of their size and scope, hold promise as vehicles for improving the control of bacterial infections, the programs have limitations. Foremost is that, even though the programs are large enough to internalize a great deal of the externalities of antibiotic use, it is unclear whether they will respond by regulating antibiotic use in a manner that minimizes costs. These are government programs, not private firms. Their managers are not rewarded for the performance or cost-effectiveness of these programs, and if the programs fail to hold down costs, they will not go out of business. Shortfalls, which are expected even for Medicare, are covered by general revenues.[19] The most direct

---

19   Duggan and Morton (2004) provide an interesting example of how poorly Medicaid controls costs and the negative impact this has on non-Medicaid consumers. Medicaid determines the price it pays for a drug by the average price for that drug in the private sector. In markets where Medicaid has a large market share of purchases, drug companies have an incentive to increase private sector prices to raise revenue from government purchases. Consistent with this prediction, Duggan and Morton find that a 10 percent increase in Medicaid market share is associated with a 10 percent increase in the private market price of a drug, holding all else constant.

evidence of this point is that neither Medicare nor Medicaid has thus far made a serious attempt to control the externalities of antibiotic use.

A second concern is that Medicare has certain large gaps in its coverage. The most obvious is that it does not include non-disabled individuals under the age of 65. Therefore it could not gather data on resistance rates or innovate on alternative therapies for this population. Another gap is its exclusion of long-term care at nursing homes. These facilities are a significant risk factor for antibiotic resistance because residents are often taking antibiotics and they also cycle through hospitals, where they often receive antibiotics. Thus, nursing homes may be pools for the emergence of resistance (Nicolle, Strausbaugh et al. 1996) and may subsequently spread resistance to hospitals. Medicaid does cover the cost of nursing homes for its enrollees. But unlike Medicare, Medicaid is neither centrally managed nor well funded. As such it has relatively less bargaining power to impose quality controls.

A third problem is that both Medicare and Medicaid are complex programs. This should be evident from the text boxes that describe the two programs (Box 6.1 and Box 6.2) as well as from the above discussion of Medicare's existing quality control programs. It is difficult enough to devise an optimal antibiotic control program, given medical uncertainty. Adding a high degree of institutional and regulatory complexity makes the problem much more challenging. The implication is not that there is no solution; there remains a second best to be achieved. Rather, the implication is that the gap between first and second best may be quite large.

## Alternative mechanisms

Medicare and, to a more limited extent, Medicaid offer unique instruments to address the problem of resistance, and it is prudent to explore their potential. They have limitations, but the extent to which these are disabling is uncertain. It may be best to attempt a series of regional but mandatory demonstration programs within Medicare to determine whether Medicare can make a difference. An important component of these efforts is to determine not just the efficacy of Medicare initiatives, but also whether failures are attributable to limitations in coverage or the nonresponsiveness of government agencies to cost incentives.

If the failures are so attributable, any game plan against resistance should consider whether private health insurance or the employers purchasing them could be employed to control resistance. For example, small employers might be allowed to pool their employees and jointly purchase insurance to increase the population coverage and thus the incentives of private insurance. Moreover, the federal or state governments might encourage employers to purchase long-term care insurance along with regular short-term care health insurance for employees to give employers an incentive to choose plans that consider the externalities in both long-term care and short-term care facilities.

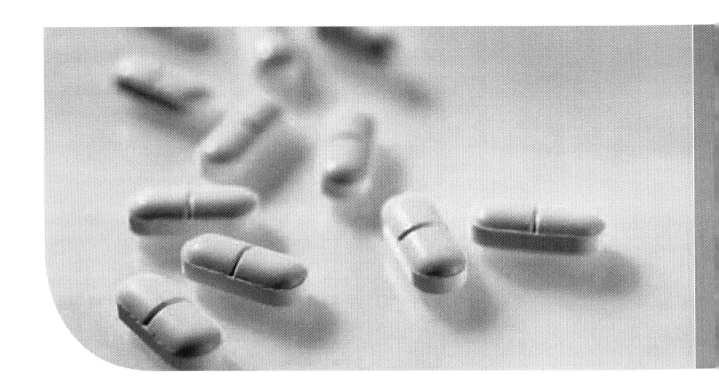

# References

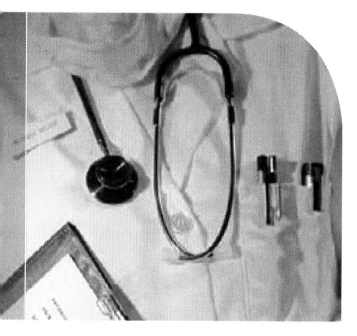

Bajaj, A. (1999). "How Medicare Calculates GME Payments, Part I." *JAMA* 281(20): 1958a.

CMS. (2005). "Fact Sheet: Physician Voluntary Reporting Program." http://www.cms.hhs.gov/apps/media/press/release.asp?Counter=1701 (accessed May 31, 2006). Centers for Medicare and Medicaid Services.

———. (2006a). "Rewarding Superior Quality Care: The Premier Hospital Quality Incentive Demonstration." http://www.cms.hhs.gov/HospitalQualityInits/downloads/HospitalPremierFS200602.pdf (accessed May 31, 2006).

———. (2006b). "Physician Voluntary Reporting Program (PVRP): 16 Measure Core Starter Set G-code Specifications and Instruction." http://www.cms.hhs.gov/PVRP/Downloads PVRPCoreStarterSet SpecificationsAndInstruction.pdf (accessed May 31, 2006).

Coase, R. H. (1960). "The Problem of Social Cost." *Journal of Law and Economics* 3: 1–44.

Cosgrove, S. E., Y. Qi, et al. (2005). "The Impact of Methicillin Resistance in *Staphylococcus aureus* Bacteremia on Patient Outcomes: Mortality, Length of Stay, and Hospital Charges." *Infection Control and Hospital Epidemiology* 26: 166–74.

Dranove, D., D. Kessler, et al. (2003). "Is More Information Better? The Effects of 'Report Cards' on Health Care Providers." *Journal of Political Economy* 111(3): 555–88.

Duggan, M., and F. S. Morton. (2004). "The Distortionary Effects of Government Procurement: Evidence from Medicaid Prescription Drug Purchasing." Working Paper 10930. Cambridge, MA: NBER (National Bureau of Economic Research.

Engemann, J. J., Y. Carmeli, et al. (2003). "Adverse Clinical and Economic Outcomes Attributable to Methicillin Resistance among Patients with *Staphylococcus aureus* Surgical Site Infection." *Clinical Infectious Diseases* 36: 592–98.

Furrow, B. R., et al. (2000). *Health Law.* 2nd ed. St. Paul, Minn.: Thomson-West.

———. (2004). *Health Law: Cases, Materials and Problems.* 5th ed. St. Paul, Minn.: Thomson-West.

Heidenreich, P. A., M. B. McClellan, et al. (2002). "The Relation between Managed Care Market Share and the Treatment of Elderly Fee-For-Service Patients with Myocardial Infarction." *The American Journal of Medicine* 112(3): 176-182.

HHS. (2006). "FAQ Sheet for NHII." http://aspe.hhs.gov/sp/NHII/FAQ.html (accessed May 31, 2006). U.S. Department of Health and Human Services.

Kaplan, R. L. (2005). "The Medicare Drug Benefit: A Prescription for Confusion." *NAELA Journal* 1(2): 167–86.

Laxminarayan, R. (2001). "Bacterial Resistance and the Optimal Use of Antibiotics." Discussion Paper 01–23. Washington, DC: Resources for the Future.

Lieberman, P. B., and M. G. Wootan. (1998). "Protecting the Crown Jewels of Medicine: A Strategic Plan to Preserve the Effectiveness of Antibiotics." http://www.cspinet.org/reports/abiotic.htm (accessed May 31, 2006).

McHugh, C. G., and W. Riley. (2004). "Risk Factors and Costs Associated with Methicillin-Resistant *Staphylococcus aureus* Bloodstream Infections." *Infection Control and Hospital Epidemiology* 25(2): 425–30.

Nicolle, L. E., L. J. Strausbaugh, et al. (1996). "Infections and Antibiotic Resistance in Nursing Homes." *Clinical Microbiology Reviews* 9(1): 1–17.

Pace, N. M., D. Golinelli, et al. (2004). "Capping Non-Economic Awards in Medical Malpractice Trials: California Jury Verdicts under MICRA." Rand Institute for Civil Justice. http://www.rand.org/publications/MG/MG234/MG234.pdf (accessed May 31, 2006).

Peters, P. G., Jr. (2002). "The Role of the Jury in Modern Malpractice Law." *Iowa Law Review* 87: 909–969.

Pittet, D., D. Tarara, et al. (1994). "Nosocomial Bloodstream Infection in Critically Ill Patients: Excess Length of Stay, Extra Costs, and Attributable Mortality." *JAMA* 271(20): 1598–601.

Pittet, D., and R. P. Wenzel. (1995). "Nosocomial Bloodstream Infections: Secular Trends in Rates, Mortality, and Contribution to Total Hospital Deaths." *Archives of Internal Medicine* 155(11): 1177–84.

Sage, W. M. (forthcoming). "The Role of Medicare in Medical Malpractice Reform." *Journal of Health Care Law & Policy* 9(2).

Smith, D. L., S. A. Levin, et al. (2005). "Strategic Interactions in Multi-Institutional Epidemics of Antibiotic Resistance." *Proceedings of the National Academy of Sciences, Early Edition.* www.pnas.org/cgi/doi/10.1073/pnas.0409523102 (accessed May 31, 2006).

Stosor, V., L. R. Peterson, et al. (1998). "*Enterococcus faecium* Bacteremia: Does Vancomycin Resistance Make a Difference?" *Archives of Internal Medicine* 158(5): 522-527.

U.S. Census Bureau. (2006). "Statistical Abstract of the United States." Washington, DC: U.S. Census Bureau.

Vidmar, N. (1995). *Medical Malpractice and the American Jury: Confronting the Myths About Jury Incompetence, Deep Pockets, and Outrageous Damage Awards.* Ann Arbor, MI: University of Michigan Press.

WSJ.com. (2006). "Key Facts. UnitedHealth Group Inc. (UNH)." http://online.wsj.com/quotes/key_facts.html?mod=2_0470&symbol=unh&news-symbol=UNH (accessed November 11, 2006). Wall Street Journal Online.

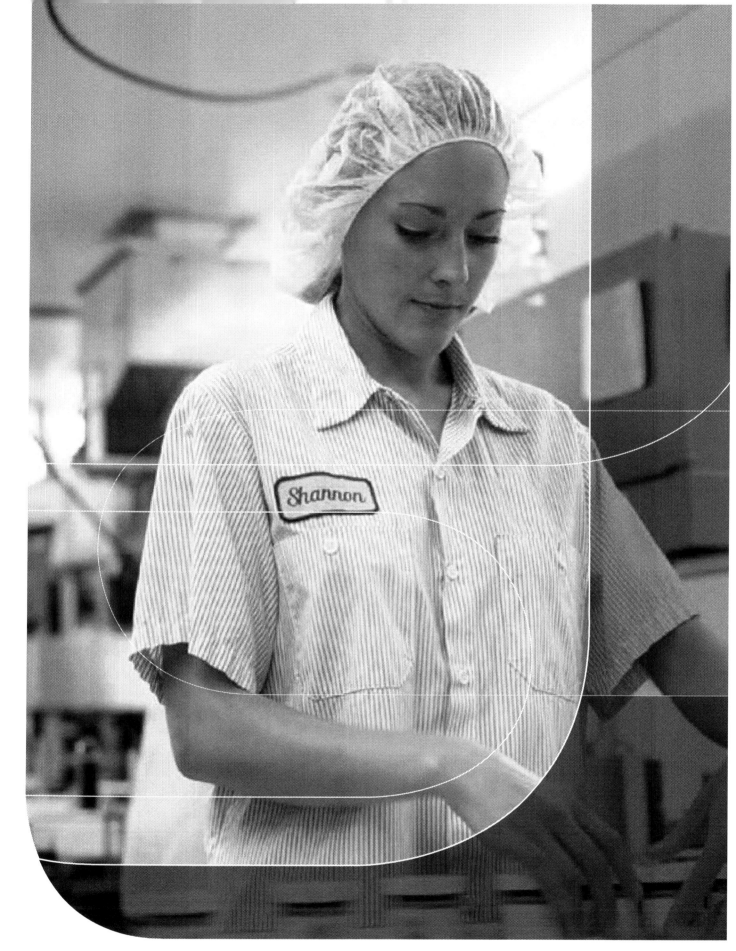

# CHAPTER 7

# Supply-side strategies for **tackling resistance**

*Anup Malani*

This chapter examines how changes in policies oriented toward suppliers of antibiotics, particularly drug companies, might be able to control antibiotic resistance. These policies include expansion of patent protection, loosening of antitrust restrictions, easing regulatory hurdles to drug approval, and rewards for the discovery of new antibiotics. Two important new lessons are, first, that there are important trade-offs between demand-side and supply-side policies. Second, solutions must be tailored to the level of the externality. For example, if use of one antibiotic generates resistance to another antibiotic, not necessarily in the same chemical class, it is important to define or permit a single property right to cover both antibiotics.

The purpose of this report is to ask how the U.S. health care system might extend the effectiveness of antibiotics. Four basic strategies are available. First, limit consumer demand for antibiotics. Second, improve the efficiency of existing antibiotics. Third, improve the rationing of antibiotics by suppliers. Fourth, develop new antibiotics. Previous chapters have focused on the first two strategies. This chapter explores the last two strategies.

The goal of the third strategy, rationing, is not to limit resistance but to allocate antibiotics to those patients who value effective antibiotics the most before resistance renders all antibiotics useless. Rationing has a cross-sectional and intertemporal component. We want to administer antibiotics to individuals who truly need them not only today (e.g., to patients with bacterial infections rather than viral infections) but also over time (e.g., to patients facing a virulent new infectious disease in the future, as opposed to patients suffering common bacterial ear infections today). Rationing can be pursued with a regulatory approach that employs practice guidelines, or with a market approach that provides incentives for drug makers to allocate antibiotics to the

> Seeking to limit demand for antibiotics or to improve the efficiency of existing antibiotics reduces the returns from finding a new antibiotic.

highest-value users. We will focus on the market incentives; chapters that address consumer demand have touched upon the regulatory approach, which includes reserving new antibiotics as drugs-of-last-resort.

The fourth strategy, developing new antibiotics, faces two hurdles. One is technological: what are the prospects of finding a new molecule or method to kill or incapacitate pathogenic bacteria? The other is behavioral: how can we get researchers and drug companies to work on overcoming the technological hurdles to a new antibiotic? Because the technological hurdles are beyond the scope of this report—policy reforms cannot change biology—we focus here on behavioral obstacles.

This chapter is organized around combating resistance by improving rationing of antibiotics and by encouraging the development of new drugs. For each strategy, we discuss the various policy levers that could be employed. With respect to rationing, the obvious levers are patent law, which grants exclusive rights to market a drug, and antitrust law, which prohibits collusion in the marketing of a drug. It will be shown that these levers address efficient rationing of on-patent antibiotics but not off-patent antibiotics. To ensure proper rationing of the latter, it may be necessary to create exclusionary rights over drugs already in the public domain. With respect to developing new antibiotics, the main lever is patent law because its main goal is to spur innovation. A

related lever is antitrust law. Patent law uses the carrot of a government monopoly to induce investment in research and development. Relaxing antitrust law, which cracks down on monopolies, might have a similar effect. Another lever is direct government support for research. The model could be research grants from the National Institutes of Health or awards like the X Prize, which seeks to encourage low-cost, private manned spaceflights.[1] Yet another lever is to relax Food and Drug Administration (FDA) standards for approval of new antibiotics. This would reduce the hurdles to marketing a new drug and thus raise the returns to its development. Particularly instructive are case studies of the Orphan Drug Act[2] and the Prescription Drug User Fee Acts,[3] whose goals were to spur new drug development. Before the analysis of the two strategies that are the topic of this chapter, however, the next two sections provide further background. Specifically, they offer guidance on comparing the four basic strategies for curbing resistance and discuss trends in the supply of new antibiotics.

■——————————————————————

## Choosing among strategies

Ultimately, readers will have to weigh not just the different tactics for rationing or improving supply but also the different strategies—demand-side and supply-side—for controlling resistance. Although the strategies are not mutually exclusive, they can undermine one another. For example, if one seeks to limit demand for antibiotics or to improve the efficiency of existing antibiotics, one is reducing the returns from—and thus the incentives for—finding a new antibiotic.[4] The reverse

---

1  See http://www.xprizefoundation.com/about_us/.

2  See http://www.fda.gov/orphan/oda.htm.

3  These comprise the Prescription Drug User Fee Act (PDUFA) of 1992, later continued as PDUFA-II in 1997 and PDUFA-III in 2002. See http://www.fda.gov/oc/pdufa/.

4  See Fidler (1998), Philipson, Rubin (2004–2005), and Mechoulan et al. (2006). The Institute of Medicine's report on antimicrobial resistance

is also true: new antibiotics reduce incentives to curb the use of or extend the life of existing antibiotics.[5]

When choosing among strategies, there are two things to keep in mind. First, limiting consumer demand for antibiotics is a "no pain, no gain" strategy. Controlling the emergence of resistant bacteria requires that consumers forgo the benefits of antibiotic use. These include improvements in the health of the patient and the positive externality of limiting the spread of drug-sensitive bacteria. In contrast, strategies that focus on the supply of existing and new antibiotics do not require this tradeoff. They offer the opportunity to forestall or defeat treatable (drug-sensitive) bacterial infections without limiting the consumption of antibiotics.

Second, there may be a way to avoid the conflict between, on the one hand, limiting demand or extending the supply of existing antibiotics and, on the other hand, generating new antibiotics. The standard tool to spur innovation is patent law. Patents give drug companies monopolies so that they can charge higher prices for new antibiotics. Efforts to curb consumer demand or bolster existing antibiotics that compete with new antibiotics will limit the prices that even monopoly producers of new antibiotics can charge. That, in turn, reduces the incentive that patents provide for the development of new antibiotics. A solution is to have the government replace private demand with its own demand for new antibiotics. This could be done by directly funding research into new antibiotics or by offering prizes for new antibiotics.

To appreciate the distinctions among the four strategies for tackling resistance, it may be useful to draw an analogy with a more familiar problem: dependence on oil. Both oil and antibiotics can be thought of as nonrenewable resources. The supply of oil is finite, and the same can be said about antibiotics: when one uses an antibiotic today, one may inadvertently encourage resistance that limits other people's use of that antibiotic tomorrow.[6] A problem with nonrenewable resources is the "tragedy of the commons" (Hardin 1968). In the oil context, if two individuals can tap the same oil deposit, they will extract and sell the oil from that deposit too quickly, since if one does not take the oil, the other will. Thus, oil is sold at the marginal cost of extraction, not at a price that reflects its limited supply. The tragedy of the commons also afflicts antibiotics. If two companies can produce the same antibiotic, each will produce and sell too many doses today for fear that, otherwise, the other company will do so and bacteria will be resistant to the antibiotic tomorrow. One solution to both problems is to assign property rights (for the oil deposit, for an antibiotic molecule) to just one individual or company. The owner of the property right should internalize the consequence of finite supply and price oil or the antibiotic so as to allocate it to the highest-value users today or tomorrow. We elaborate on this connection further below.[7]

---

acknowledges this in the context of calls for FDA to condition approval for antibiotics on restriction on use (Harrison and Lederberg 1998). Industry sources also blame demand controls for limited supplies (Service 2004).

5   A related problem is that development of one new antibiotic reduces demand for a second new antibiotic more than in the ordinary case, where a new brand of widget reduces demand for existing brands of widgets. The reason is that a new antibiotic actually shifts the demand curve for all new antibiotics back toward the origin. The shift occurs because the new antibiotic lowers the probability of resistance to any given antibiotic. Even if a bacterium develops resistance to an existing antibiotic, the new antibiotic will kill it (Ellison and Hellerstein 1999).

6   In a previous chapter it is suggested that antibiotic effectiveness may be renewable. Because resistance has a fitness cost, it may be possible to "renew" an antibiotic by not using it for a period. During this period, nonresistant strains of bacteria may be reintroduced and, because of the fitness costs of resistance, outcompete resistant strains. Once nonresistant strains eliminate resistant strains, antibiotics will once again be useful. Nonetheless, there are two reasons to treat antibiotic effectiveness as a nonrenewable resource. First, it may take some time for nonresistant strains to return. In the short run, therefore, antibiotic effectiveness may be presumed finite. Second, when resistant strains die out, they may leave fragments of their DNA, which encode their mechanism for resistance, in the host's bloodstream. When antibiotics are used, nonresistant strains may pick up resistance not just from mutations, but also from scavenging DNA fragments in the bloodstream. As a result, after the renewal period, nonresistant strains may acquire resistance much faster than before that period. In short, renewal may eke out only a little more antibiotic resistance. When the cost of the nonuse period is factored in, the returns to renewal may be very limited.

7   A second level at which oil consumption is analogous to antibiotic use

Both the common pool problem and the pollution externality for oil have led to calls for policy reforms that resemble the four strategies for tackling resistance. One is to curb use of oil: energy conservation. The most common tactic is a gas tax. Another strategy is to extract more energy from or limit the pollution emitted from any fixed amount of oil. The usual policy levers are corporate average fuel economy (CAFE) standards and emissions limits. A third strategy might be to ration oil. This strategy has been employed to stop the common pool resource problems with oil deposits, but not to limit pollution from oil consumption. The last strategy is to develop new oil deposits and alternative sources of energy. This is implemented via tax breaks for exploration and for alternative fuels or technologies that use alternative fuels. The way in which policymakers choose among these different strategies for combating dependence on oil can guide their choice among the strategies for combating resistance.

## Trends in the supply of new antibiotics

It is difficult to determine the future supply of new antibiotics. Statistical evidence suggests that the rate of innovation is lagging, yet many analysts blame this lack of innovation on the lack of substantial aggregate demand for new antibiotics. If demand is the culprit, however, then it is possible that, if aggregate demand increases then so might supply. To put it in economic terms, all one can identify when one looks at trends in investment in or applications for the approval of new antibiotics is the intersection of the aggregate demand and supply curves for new antibiotics at recent levels of demand. One cannot determine what the future supply will be, given a change—presumably a large increase—in

the aggregate demand for new antibiotics. Innovation may accelerate to meet a future increase in demand because of the emergence of resistance against older antibiotics. Perhaps this optimism is unwarranted: after all, some analysts suggest that innovation takes a long time, perhaps a decade or more (Tanouye 1996; Gilcrest 2004).[8] But delays in research and development are only a concern if future increases in demand cannot be predicted. The problem for policymaking, then, is that we do not know the probability with which resistance and thus the demand for new antibiotics will unexpectedly and dramatically rise. The aim here is not to encourage readers to be optimistic about the future, but to acknowledge how little we know. With that caveat, let us turn to the data we do have.

By most accounts, the rate of innovation in antibiotics slowed in the 1980s (Travis 1994). After a series of professional conferences that sounded an alarm over resistance and highlighted the deceleration of innovation (*Science* 1994; Tanouye 1996), research and development picked up. The results, however, have been less than spectacular. Figure 7.1 graphs the number of new antibacterial agents approved in the United States between 1983 and 2005. The decline in new approvals has been both consistent and dramatic: from 16 in 1983–1987 to 7 in 1998–2002 (Spellberg, Powers et al. 2004).[9] Since then, only 4 new antibiotics have been approved (Bosso 2005). Looking forward, the picture is not much more promising. There are only 12

---

is that both have externalities. An important distinction, however, is that whereas oil consumption has a negative externality (pollution), antibiotic use has a positive externality (reducing the spread of antibiotic-susceptible bacterial infections). (The negative externality from antibiotic use does not have a distinct effect from the tragedy of the commons problem that afflicts antibiotic use.)

8  For example, the Tufts Center for Drug Development (2001) estimates it takes 10 to 15 years to bring a drug from discovery to approval for sale in the United States. This estimate is a range for all drugs, not just antibiotics.

9  For comparison, note that 225 total new molecular entities were approved by FDA from 1998 to 2002. Thus only 3 percent (7 of 225) were antibacterials. To be fair, however, it should be acknowledged that the decline in approval of new drugs is not unique to antibiotics. Submissions of new molecular entities for FDA approval fell from nearly 45 in 1996 to 25 in 2003 (FDA 2004, Figure 2). Moreover, it has been alleged that many of the drugs approved in the 1980s and 1990s were not more effective than placebos or existing drugs. If one controls for such efficacy, there may be no discernible trend in uniquely *effective* antibiotic approvals.

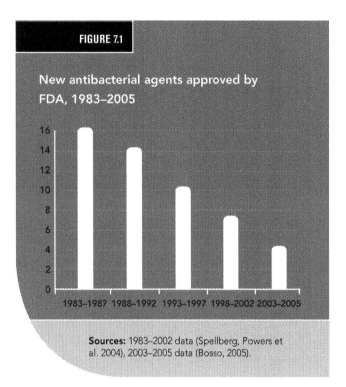

**FIGURE 7.1**

New antibacterial agents approved by FDA, 1983–2005

Sources: 1983–2002 data (Spellberg, Powers et al. 2004), 2003–2005 data (Bosso, 2005).

What makes matters worse is that few of these NMEs employ a novel mechanism of action. This is important because a molecule with a novel mechanism may delay the time until resistance emerges: the evolutionary adaptive response that bacteria must make to a novel mechanism is, in probabilistic terms, much more dramatic than that to an existing mechanism. A good analogy is how easily a seasoned basketball player would adjust to a change in the location of the three-point line versus how much he would have to change to play a new game, like baseball. Of the 9 new antimicrobials approved between 1998 and 2003, only 2 have novel mechanisms (Spellberg, Powers et al. 2004, Table 1). Of the 12 antimicrobials beyond phase 1 studies but not yet approved, only 2 have novel mechanisms (Talbot, Bradley et al. 2006, Table 2).

Although this picture is grim, the situation may not be as dire as the raw statistics suggest. First, many of the antibiotics currently in the research pipeline target MRSA, an important health risk (measured in aggregate dollar cost). Indeed, if the antibacterial molecules that are currently awaiting FDA approval join those recently approved, we may have several new options, and MRSA may no longer be considered as serious a mortality risk as it is now. Balanced against this is the lack of new drug development to address the untreatable infections caused by Gram-negative bacteria, such as *Escherichia coli*, *Acinetobacter baumannii*, *Enterobacter*, *Klebsiella pneumoniae*, and *Pseudomonas aeruginosa*.

Second, antibiotics are an important complement to many new medical technologies, including surgical procedures, implanted medical devices, and immuno-suppressive drugs for cancer.[13] A common side effect of these technologies is

antimicrobial compounds beyond phase 1 studies but not yet approved by FDA (Talbot, Bradley et al. 2006, Table 2).[10] Furthermore, only a tiny fraction of new molecular entities (NMEs) in drug companies' publicly disclosed research and development programs are antibacterials. Among the world's 15 largest pharmaceutical companies, only 5 of 315 NMEs are antibacterials. At the 7 largest biotechnology companies, only 1 of 81 NMEs is an antibacterial (Spellberg, Powers et al. 2004).[11] Importantly, none of the above molecules specifically target Gram-negative bacteria.[12]

---

10 There are also 5 antifungals and 6 antistaphylococcal vaccines or immunoglobulins (Talbot, Bradley et al. 2006, Tables 1 and 3).

11 Recent reports by the Infectious Diseases Society of America (IDSA 2004; Talbot, Bradley et al. 2006) offer more detailed information on which new antibiotics are being developed for specific bacterial species (*Acinetobacter baumannii*, *Aspergillus*, ESBL-producing *Escherichia coli* and *Klebsiella pneumoniae*, *Pseudomonas aeruginosa*, VRE, and MRSA).

12 Some antibiotic molecules are wide spectrum. And some antibiotics targeted toward Gram-positive bacteria can be combined with drugs that break down the cell walls of Gram-negative bacteria. Nevertheless, we are

---

further behind in research on Gram-negative strains than on Gram-positive strains.

13 Antibiotics are also a complement to many existing medical technologies. Therefore, an important positive externality from improving antibiotic efficacy, whether accomplished by reducing use or by developing new antibiotics, is to improve the productivity of these medical technologies.

that they place treated patients at greater risk for bacterial infections. As more and more of these technologies emerge, there will be more demand for antibiotics, including new molecules with activity against resistant bacterial strains. This will naturally increase the return to new antibiotic development in the future.

Third, there are some promising signs on the scientific front, including research on bacteriophages, viruses that attack bacteria (Martin 2003). (This class of treatment also includes gene therapies that are administered with viruses; Cromie 2001.) Commonly used in the former Soviet bloc countries, these viruses are only now being developed in the West (Box 7.1). A phage-based antibiotic to treat *Listeria monocytogenes* in poultry was granted an experimental use permit by the Environmental Protection Agency in June 2002. But phages targeting human infections are far from obtaining FDA approval (Martin 2003). Another promising avenue of research is inhibiting the quorum-sensing ability of bacteria (Box 7.2). Certain bacteria are capable of sensing their own population density so as to optimally time their attacks or to set up defenses. If this ability could be thwarted, bacteria would be rendered less harmful or more susceptible to antibiotics.

Four itemized market factors, industry analysts suggest, are responsible for the recent lack of innovation on antimicrobials (Spellberg, Powers et al. 2004). The first is the large number of existing antibiotics, which are competitors of any new antibiotic. More than 100 antimicrobials have already been approved in the United States (Bartlett, Auwaerter et al. 2007). And a majority of bacterial infections are still caused by bacteria susceptible to existing antibiotics (Powers 2004). Even if a new drug is granted a patent, it will not be able to charge supracompetitive prices to recoup research and

development costs because of these competitors. (The corollary is that when existing antibiotics fail, as in the case of MRSA, there is targeted and successful innovation.) Second, doctors tend to "reserve" new antibiotics until existing antibiotics are rendered ineffective by resistance (see also Rubin 2004–2005). Reserving delays the use of antibiotics. Even if the delay does not push the new antibiotic into the period when the developer's patent has expired, it will delay the date when the drug will begin making profits. Third, a related concern among drug companies is that doctors tend to avoid new antibiotics because of their high price tags. Doctors often have the interest of not just their patients' health but also their (or their payers') pocketbooks in mind when choosing medications. They will choose a lower-priced drug if it is nearly equally effective. This too reduces the return to companies from development of new antibiotics. Fourth, drug companies prefer to focus on treatments for chronic diseases, for market reasons. The U.S. population is aging, and older people are more likely to have chronic conditions than acute infections requiring antibiotics.[14] Moreover, patients with chronic ailments continually purchase treatment for these ailments, providing drug companies a steady source of revenue. Effective antibiotics, however, require only one course of treatment: patients are not repeat customers for the same ailment (see also Service 2004).[15]

---

14  That said, bacterial infections often complicate chronic conditions, such as diabetes or HIV (Stinson 1996). Effective antibiotics can therefore be thought of as a useful complement to treatments for chronic conditions.

15  An analogy for the diminished incentive that drug companies have to produce antibiotics may be the diminished incentive monopolists have to produce truly durable goods. If the monopolist produces a truly durable good, present sales compete against future sales. Unless the monopolist can commit to a future price schedule or rent for its durable product, it will not be able to extract supracompetitive profits (Coase 1972). This analogy has been explored in the context of vaccine production (Kremer and Snyder 2004; Forslid 2006). But one weakness in this analogy is that patients cannot delay their consumption of an antibiotic as they can for, say, light bulbs. If patients cannot delay consumption, then future sales may not compete with existing sales.

---

Because this externality is probably not fully internalized by those seeking to control use of antibiotics or researching new ones, there is likely insufficient investment in promoting antibiotic effectiveness.

## BACTERIOPHAGES

Bacteriophages, or "bacteria eaters," were first reported as far back as 1896, but it was not until 1917 that they were identified and named by a French Canadian bacteriologist, Felix d'Herelle (Martin 2003). Bacteriophages, or phages for short, are viruses that attack bacteria. A phage has a large modular head in which it carry its genes, a tunnellike tail, and long, reedy legs used to attach to the bacterium (see image). The phage uses its tail to bore a hole into the bacterium and inject its genes. Once inside, the genes force the host into constructing new phages until the bacterium actually bursts apart, releasing hundreds of new phages (Radetsky 1996).

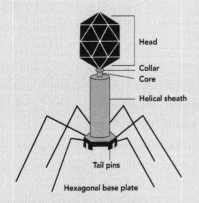

The promise of phages is that they are one of the most abundant life forms on the planet and readily available in the environment, and unlike antibiotics, they replicate themselves: a patient would not need repeated doses. They also have evolved to target specific bacteria, avoiding many of the complications associated with antibiotics, such as adverse reactions or the destruction of "good" bacteria, and they can mutate, which allows them to genetically evolve with the bacteria, thus reducing the likelihood of resistance. This is why d'Herelle proposed that these viruses could function as "our friend" and energetically promoted them, and in the ensuing years, phage therapy was used extensively around the world. But with the discovery of penicillin in the 1940s, research and use in the western world stopped, though it continued in Tbilisi, Georgia, at an institute that d'Herelle helped found. During that time, Russian scientists created treatments for everything from dysentery to blood poisoning to urinary tract infections, and in at least one case phages have been used as a prophylaxis (Radetsky 1996). Yet much of the research from this time period is inaccessible or classified (Braun 2006).

Today, the future of phage technology is being revived in the West; phages are being developed to destroy pathogens that infect domestic farm production animals and their environment, including aqua farms, and have also been proposed to fight bacterial infections of crops, such as citrus canker (Levin and Bull 2004). However, their greatest promise is human drug development, where advances in the biology and genetic understanding of phages (Campbell 2003) and the ability to genetically engineer phages (Westwater and Kasman 2003) have biotechnology firms racing to bring phage therapy to market as an alternative or supplement to antibiotics. Animal studies have so far proven successful (Bull, Levin et al. 2002), and although FDA has begun establishing criteria for the approval process and reviewing applications for physician investigational drug trials, which were expected to begin in late 2006 (Sulakvelidze 2006), there are still many questions that surround the efficacy and safety of phages. Actual approval of human drugs is still years away (Schoolnik, Summers et al. 2004).

—Eili Klein

**BOX 7.2**

## QUORUM SENSING

It has long been appreciated that certain groups of bacteria are capable of interacting with each other and their surrounding environment through the use of chemical signals. Of particular interest is a specific form of cell-to-cell communication that allows bacteria to detect their own population density and express genes based on this, a method termed quorum sensing (Fuqua, Winans et al. 1994). Each species has different means of communicating, but in general, the bacteria produce a signal molecule that begins to build up in the surrounding environment. Once a specific threshold level is met, the molecule binds to and activates a receptor protein on the bacteria. The activated receptor then expresses or inhibits certain genes, which alter the bacteria cell and can induce several behaviors, including attacking the host and its production of defense mechanisms (Williams 2006). For example, *Pseudomonas aeruginosa*, a deadly human pathogen, is especially virulent because of its ability to secrete toxins, enzymes, and proteins that destroy and degrade human cells. However, the expression of these harmful exoproducts does not occur until the density of the bacteria is high (Albus, Pesci et al. 1997).

The promise of quorum sensing lies in the possibility that infections could be controlled by inhibiting the quorum-sensing capabilities of bacteria. Generally, three main avenues of approach have been recognized as points to attack the ability of bacteria to communicate: 1) blocking the production of the signal molecule; 2) inactivating or destroying the signal molecules; and 3) interfering with the receptor so as to inhibit detection of the signal molecule. Since none of these approaches interfere with or directly impede the processes of the bacteria that are essential for growth, they may not produce the harsh conditions that lead to selective pressure and resistance, as antibiotics do (Rasmussen and Givskov 2006).

Promising results have been obtained in both degrading the signal molecule and interfering with the signal receptor. In both cases, the natural world has provided clues as to how to proceed, since bacteria have been found that produce an enzyme that breaks down the signal molecule of other bacteria. And in plant trials, genetic manipulation of colonizing bacteria to express this defense was able to prevent the infection of the plant by virulent bacteria. Fungi and plants also produce a set of compounds that can inactivate the signal molecule or inhibit the signal receptor. In a promising development, these compounds, though not able to completely inhibit the quorum sensing of bacteria, have been able to attenuate the virulence of the infections, with pronounced effects on mortality (Rasmussen and Givskov 2006).

Despite the promising laboratory studies, the ability to block quorum sensing and thus control bacterial infections has not been established to work effectively in the complex environment of a living organism, and thus it will likely be years before effective treatments based on quorum sensing begin to appear.

—Eili Klein

Despite those disincentives for investment in antibiotic development, the market for antibiotics appears to be large and growing. Anti-infectives (which include antibiotics and antivirals) are the third-largest therapeutic area in terms of worldwide sales (Bush 2004, Table 4). According to BCC Research (2001), the total global market for antibiotics will cross $34.5 billion in 2006. The demand for new antibiotics in particular will be $7.4 billion and is expected to grow at an annual rate of 34 percent (Gray 2004).[16] This information is not new: even a decade ago, analysts suggested that a breakthrough antibiotic could be worth more than $1 billion per year in worldwide sales (Tanouye 1996).

■

## Rationing existing antibiotics

Nonrenewable resources, whether oil or antibiotics, are subject to the tragedy of the commons. There are many solutions to the tragedy of the commons. Hardin (1968) stressed government regulation of consumption. Ellickson (1986) has highlighted a role for customs or traditions. But economists starting with Gordon (1954) and Coase (1960) have tended to focus on market solutions, specifically the use of property rights. If the government gives property rights over the oil deposit to one person or company, that actor will consider the opportunity cost of forgone future extraction and sale when it decides whether to extract and sell the oil today—an observation Hotelling made in a famous 1931 article on exhaustible resources. The result will be an efficient rate of extraction of the oil over time.[17]

Because an oil deposit is attached to surrounding land, defining property rights simply requires enforcing rights over access to that land. If a deposit overlaps multiple parcels of land, the law need merely permit an individual to purchase and merge the multiple parcels under her ownership.[18] Antibiotics, however, are not attached to any physical entity over which traditional property rights may be assigned. If one company produces one pill of a given antibiotic, what stops another from producing another pill of the same antibiotic? Under the current legal regime in the United States, patent law gives the owner of an antibiotic patent the exclusive right to produce the drug for sale.[19]

## :: THE ROLE OF PATENTS

Patent law is intended not to solve a commons problem but to encourage innovation.[20] As a result, there is a poor

for the antibiotic over which property rights are properly defined, then competition among the antibiotics will eliminate the monopoly pricing effect. In addition, the owner of the property right may use the monopoly rents to engage in more research and development than would occur in the case where there are no or incomplete property rights over the antibiotic. In that case, there is a dynamic benefit to the monopoly rents that offsets some of the costs from inefficiently low overall supply of the antibiotic.

18 An alternative to pooling the plots under one owner is to craft a unitization agreement that pools not the land but the oil revenues from all plots. The agreement then allocates these revenues across plot owners according to some measure, such as the volume of oil under each plot. This revenue sharing discourages the common pool problem by eliminating the benefits a plot owner obtains from extracting oil beyond his plot (or share of revenues). See Kim and Mahoney (2005).

19 See Brown and Gruben (1997), who argue generically that intellectual property rights can help promote preservation of product effectiveness.

20 Edmund Kitch (1977) has proposed that patent law is also intended to encourage the commercialization of an innovation—that is, investment in turning an idea into a usable product and advertising that product for sale. These activities, like innovation, are public goods that would not be optimally supplied without property rights protection. This "prospect" theory of patents intends a related but distinct role for patent law different from that discussed in this chapter. Prospect theory focuses on taking an innovation from idea to consumption. Here we consider using patent law to encourage the owner of an innovation, even after commercialization, to ration production so as to account for intertemporal consumption externalities. For antibiotics, which are like nonrenewable resources, the externality is that one person's consumption reduces the efficacy of another person's consumption.

16 In addition, there are some developmental advantages antibiotics have over drugs in other therapeutic classes. It is easier to predict whether they will be successful, they have well-defined biomarkers, clinical trials are shorter, and because the duration of therapy is shorter, there is less risk of side effects (Bush 2004; Powers 2004).

17 An important side effect of the property rights approach is that it may lead to monopoly pricing if one company is given control over an antibiotic and there are no therapeutic substitutes for that antibiotic. The result will be inefficiently low overall consumption of antibiotics (even though there will be efficient allocation of this limited consumption of the antibiotic over time and consumers). If there are antibiotics that are therapeutic substitutes

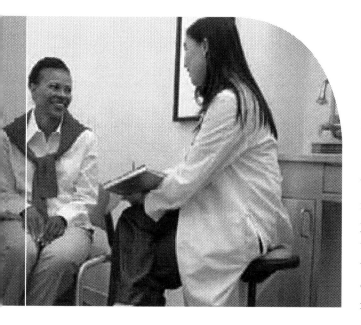

to different chemical classes.[21] Patent law, however, may assign distinct patents to two different antibiotics within any one functional group. For example, Pfizer has a patent over extended-release azithromycin (Zithromax), and Abbott has a patent over extended-release clarithromycin (Biaxin XL). Both happen to be members of the macrolide chemical class of antibiotics. This means that even though sales of Zithromax by Pfizer may reduce the efficacy of Biaxin XL by Abbott, Pfizer and Abbott have exclusive use of their respective antibiotics.[22] One solution is for Pfizer to sell its patent rights over Zithromax to Abbott, or vice versa. But that may raise antitrust problems, which we address later in this chapter.[23] Another solution is to define patent rights not over any specific antibiotic but over all antibiotics within a functional resistance group (Laxminarayan 2001).[24]

fit between the current structure of patent law and the sort of structure necessary to avoid the commons problem with antibiotic use. For one thing, patents have limited duration. In nominal terms it is 20 years. Given the legal requirement and the time necessary to obtain FDA approval before marketing a new drug, the effective duration of a patent may be much less. One solution, proposed by Kades (2005), is to give patents over antibiotics an effectively infinite duration.

But that leaves a second issue: resistance externalities across patentable antibiotics. To analyze this issue, it is helpful to categorize antibiotics into groups not as they are currently done (by chemical classes, such as macrolides or fluoroquinolones) but based on the extent to which they trigger resistance that is also effective against other antibiotics. For clarity we shall call groups of antibiotics based on this categorization "functional (resistance) groups" or simply groups. A detailed description of the categorization may be found in Box 2.1, in Chapter 2. This categorization is useful because two antibiotics within a functional group are more likely to have negative resistance externalities on each other, even though they may belong

21  In truth, any antibiotic can have a resistance externality on any other. However, the probability or seriousness of the externality rises when the two antibiotics share the same mechanism of action. In other words, the resistance externality across antibiotics is more severe within functional resistance groups, as we have defined them, than across these groups. We focus only on controlling externalities within groups because property rights also convey monopoly powers, and greater monopoly power generates potentially greater deadweight loss due to pricing. Within groups, the resistance externality may be significant enough to justify creating property rights over the entire group despite the monopoly risks. Across groups, however, the danger from externalities is not severe enough to warrant incurring the monopoly costs from creating a single property right over all antibiotics.

22  It is not obvious that the externality will always be negative. If two companies each develop an antibiotic within the same functional group, but the second is designed to overcome resistance to the first, greater production of the first antibiotic will increase demand for the second antibiotic. Whether the externality is positive or negative, however, defining property rights over the group will yield a more optimal level of rationing.

23  An advantage that patent pools have over defining broader patent rights is that the composition of the pools can change over time. This is valuable because the composition of functional resistance groups may change over time as bacteria develop new mechanisms for resisting an antibiotic. These new mechanisms may not work against certain other members of the same, preexisting functional group, and it may work against antibiotics not in the current group. We suspect that private licensing arrangements will be more flexible and responsive to these evolutionary adjustments than government allocations of patent rights.

24  A useful consequence—though one that does not motivate our proposal—of extending patent length and width would be to encourage

Even that is an incomplete solution, however, because many groups of antibiotics already exist that have either member antibiotics without patent protection or different member antibiotics whose patents are held by different companies. If a functional resistance group contains an antibiotic without patent protection, anyone can produce it. There is no way to stop the externalities from that production. If a group contains multiple patents held by different companies, again, some entity has to buy up all the patents in the group, raising antitrust problems.

A solution to the off-patent problem could be the creation of a *sui generis* ("of its own kind") right. Such a right may borrow some of the features of a right granted under patent law but does not have a basis in patent law or draw authority from the intellectual property clause in the U.S. Constitution.[25] A *sui generis* right must be adopted by Congress and may be justified by reliance on some other enumerated power of Congress, such as that granted in the commerce clause (Nachbar 2004). *Sui generis* rights are typically proposed to fill gaps in existing systems of rights. These rights have been proposed and occasionally adopted to protect semiconductor designs, databases, and biodiversity. To address the off-patent problem, a *sui generis* right over an off-patent antibiotic would borrow from patent law the feature that only the holder could produce the covered antibiotic.[26] For the reasons given above, the right should be perpetual, and the rights over all off-patent antibiotics from a given functional resistance group of antibiotics should be assigned to the same company or individual. (Different groups of off-patent antibiotics, however, could be assigned to different companies or individuals.)

---

innovation in antibacterials. But for reasons given later, the effect on innovation may not be very large.

25  Art. I, Sec. 8 reads, in part, "The Congress shall have Power... To promote the Progress of Science and useful Arts, by securing for limited Times to Authors and Inventors the exclusive Right to their respective Writings and Discoveries."

26  What we are proposing, in other words, is a right over a currently open-access resource, viz. off-patent drugs.

The difficult question raised by a *sui generis* right over off-patent antibiotics concerns to whom the right should be assigned. The only recent example in which the U.S. government has granted a monopoly over an off-patent technology is the Orphan Drug Act (21 U.S.C. §§ 360aa–ee), which grants a seven-year period of marketing exclusivity (§360cc) for any drug, whether on patent or off, that can be used to treat an ailment that affects 200,000 or fewer persons (§360bb(a)(2)). That statute assigns the monopoly right to the company that demonstrates the efficacy of the drug for the rare disease. This is not possible with a *sui generis* right over off-patent antibiotics because anyone can demonstrate the efficacy of each antibiotic for an array of ailments. One solution may be to simply hold an auction over rights to production. An analogy would be the 1993 amendments to the Telecommunications Act of 1934 (47 U. S. C. §309(j)(1)), which, along with Federal Communications Commission regulations (e.g., In re-implementation of Section 309(j) of the Communications Act—Competitive Bidding, 9 FCC Rcd. 2348, ¶¶54, 68 (1994)), authorized the auction of radio spectrum to the highest bidders. An advantage of this approach would be that the government could extract any supracompetitive rents that the *sui generis* right might generate. Whatever the method chosen to assign *sui generis* rights over off-patent antibiotics, companies that currently produce generic versions of covered antibiotics may protest the closing of their business. They are unlikely to prevail in court, however, because it has long been settled that the government needs only to provide a "rational basis" to be allowed by courts to grant an exclusive right over off-patent technology (*Evans v. Jordan* 1813; Epstein 2002, 142). In this case, the possibility that *sui generis* rights may help control resistance externalities is that basis. Courts are therefore likely to side with the government and reject the complaints of generics manufacturers.

Even if broader and longer patents can handle externalities across future antibiotics and analogous *sui generis* rights can handle externalities across off-patent antibiotics, how is one to address resistance across antibiotics that are currently on patent? These patents could be revoked, and whatever exclusive production and marketing rights they included could be bundled into *sui generis* rights or any future grant of broad antibiotic group patents. Because current patent holders have a property interest in their patented technology, however, the government would have to compensate the patent holders for their lost profits under the takings clause of the Fifth Amendment. If the government raised enough money by auctioning off *sui generis* rights, it might be able to afford this compensation. But given that off-patent antibiotics are much more likely to already suffer from resistance, those auctions are unlikely to raise sufficient revenue. A second problem is that revoking a legitimate patent is an unprecedented act and therefore may not be politically feasible. An alternative solution is to rely on patent holders within a functional group to sell their patents to a single company. Again, antitrust law may get in the way. Moreover,

depending on one's faith in the market, one might have more or less confidence that private actors would consolidate all patents within a group (and only within a group).

Imagine if one were to overcome those hurdles. Table 7.1 summarizes policy proposals for addressing resistance externalities across hypothetical antibiotics by three types of patent status. Yet what are we to do about resistance externalities across antibiotics of different patent statuses? The answer is the same as in the previous paragraph. Extending either *sui generis* rights or future patents over all antibiotics regardless of patent status would entail a takings that would require just compensation. The alternative is to rely on licensing agreements that consolidate rights over all antibiotics from a functional resistance group, regardless of patent status, in one company (last row of Table 7.1). Consolidation, however, raises antitrust questions, to which we now turn.

## :: THE ANTITRUST ISSUE

Ideally, under the "rule of reason" in U.S. antitrust cases, evaluation of the consolidation of all antibiotics within a functional group in one company should depend only on the net effect on efficiency. Simply put, the consolidation would have to meet only two conditions to pass scrutiny. First, it would have to promote economic efficiency. That is, consolidation must have some social benefit and not just redistribute wealth to producers. The resistance externalities should satisfy this condition. Second, the company must not have sufficient market power to raise the average market price of the antibiotic group. (It could raise the current price but lower the future price by implicitly shifting supply from current consumers to future consumers through rationing, but it could not raise the average for a dose across time.) The purpose of this condition is to ensure that the consolidation is used only to promote efficiency and not to generate supracompetitive rents. Although it is difficult to determine the effect of consolidation on market price, an indirect measure is to determine the effect that consolidation has on

| Table 7.1 | POLICY SOLUTIONS TO RESISTANCE EXTERNALITIES | | |
|---|---|---|---|
| PATENT STATUS | HYPOTHETICAL ANTIBIOTICS FROM A GIVEN FUNCTIONAL RESISTANCE GROUP OF ANTIBIOTICS | | HORIZONTAL SOLUTION |
| Off-patent antibiotic | Antibiotic 1, Company A | Antibiotic 2, Company B | Perpetual *sui generis* right over both antibiotics auctioned to one company |
| Currently patented antibiotic | Antibiotic 3, Company C | Antibiotic 4, Company D | Antitrust exemption to allow sale of both antibiotics to one company |
| Future antibiotic | Antibiotic 5, Company E | Antibiotic 6, Company F | Broader, perpetual patent right covering entire group of new antibiotics |
| Vertical solution | Antitrust exemption to allow sale of *sui generis* and patent rights to one company | | |

the market share of the relevant group of antibiotics. A court might define the market narrowly to include only a specific ailment, such as staph infections, or broadly to include an array of bacteria. Regardless, there are two questions: how many other groups of antibiotics compete in that market, and what is the market share of the defendant's group? If the implied Herfindahl-Hirschman Index over market shares for competing functional groups is sufficiently low,[27] then the second condition will be met. To summarize, if one functional group of antibiotics competes with a sufficient number of other such groups of antibiotics, consolidation will be allowed. (If markets are defined narrowly, this analysis will be repeated for each relevant bacterial infection. If, on balance, the efficiencies from managing resistance outweigh the inefficiencies from market concentration across markets, the consolidation should be permitted.) If this condition is not met, the consolidation will be prosecuted as either a contract in restraint of trade under Section 1 of the Sherman Act, 15 U.S.C. §1, or as an attempt to monopolize under

Section 2 of that act. It is less than obvious that the efficiencies will favor consolidation. But if they do not, perhaps it is not worth controlling resistance in the first place (at least through consolidation).

Unfortunately, consolidation of patents might not be evaluated under the rule of reason. Courts might not understand the resistance externality, be able to analyze the bacterial markets in which antibiotics compete, or trust private firms with rationing to control resistance. Worse, instead of analogizing to the case of vertical arrangements between complementary products (complementary because of the externalities), the courts might analogize to the case of horizontal arrangements (horizontal because antibiotics within a functional group may compete with one another). More precisely, courts might rule that patent holders' selling all patents to one company accomplishes the same result as patent holders' simply colluding to set prices or divide markets for their patents. Continuing the logic, because collusion is per se illegal under *U.S. v. Socony-Vacuum Oil Co.* (1940), so is consolidation.

What is the implication? Because the rule of reason may not apply to—let alone protect—consolidation, it would likely be necessary for Congress to carve an exception to antitrust enforcement against consolidation of antibiotic

---

27   The Herfindahl-Hirschman Index (HHI) is the sum of squared market shares of functional groups. Here, market shares are defined by bacterial infection and context (outpatient, inpatient, surgical site, lung, blood, etc.), not antibiotic or antibiotic group. The minimum HHI is zero, and the maximum is one. The higher the HHI, the higher the degree of market concentration and thus market power.

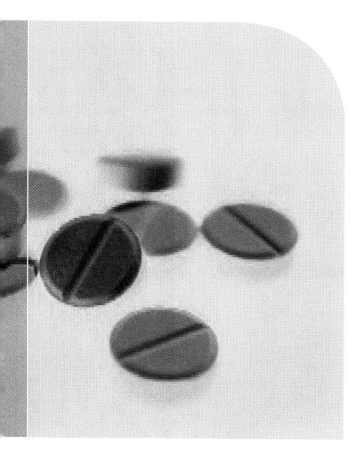

resistance groups rather than individual antibiotics. One heretofore ignored complication is health insurance. Private rationing is implemented through pricing. If the owner of an antibiotic group wants to reserve an antibiotic for a future use, then it sets the current price to a level, adjusted for the time value of money, that it thinks a future consumer would pay for that antibiotic. Any patients who value current consumption more than that level will be able to purchase a dose from the class. But if patients have health insurance, they may be insensitive to price and consume a dose today even though they do not value it at the price that the owner of the group has set. Thus health insurance may defeat private rationing via the price mechanism.[28] Another complication is that resistant bacteria travel across borders. Even if the United States were to restructure its property rights and antitrust laws to control resistance externalities across antibiotics, resistant bacterial strains may develop outside our borders in countries that have not acted to address these externalities. Those strains may spread to the United States via air travelers or commercial shippers. This would reduce the return to our own efforts at controlling resistance externalities. One solution is to seek to harmonize, by treaty, the property right and antitrust rules governing antibiotics across countries. This is no small task, but it may be an essential complement to the policy proposals developed in this section.

■

## Stimulating new antibiotics

:: PATENT OPTIONS

An alternative to rationing existing antibiotics is to create new antibiotics, especially those that have novel mechanisms of action and thus constitute new functional groups of antibiotics. The primary mechanism to encourage such

patents within a functional resistance group. Models for the exemption include those for agricultural cooperatives (Capper-Volstead Agricultural Producers' Associations Act, 7 U.S.C. §§ 291–292), unions (Section 6, Clayton Act, 15 U.S.C. § 17), or certain joint operations among newspapers (Newspaper Preservation Act of 1970, 15 U.S.C. §§ 1801–1804). The downside is that, whether the decision is to usurp existing patent rights and pay compensation or to allow private, voluntary consolidation of patents, congressional authorization—no small hurdle—will be required.

Before turning to the strategy of stimulating the supply of new antibiotics, consider two more caveats to the strategy of rationing by assigning property rights over functional

---

28   That said, health insurance companies may have their own reasons and tools to control resistance. We explored these in Chapter 6.

innovation is patent law. Patent law gives the patent holder the right to bar other entities from producing for consumption or marketing a patented antibiotic. At a minimum, this right prevents other entities from free-riding on a company's innovation. In other words, it allows a company to internalize the benefits of its investment in research and development.

Internalization, however, generates investment only in proportion to the market power a patent holder possesses. If two patented antibiotics equally treat the same ailment, however, neither patent holder will be able to capture much in the way of supracompetitive profits. But it is these profits that motivate (and fund) investment in innovation. Thus patent law will do little to spur innovation where there are "dueling patents." Nor will a patent create much incentive to develop new antibiotics where that antibiotic has to compete with existing, off-patent antibiotics. Unfortunately, there are currently numerous on- and off-patent antibiotics to compete with almost any new antibiotics.

So the question becomes, is there any way to generate market power so as to stimulate investment through patent law? For obvious reasons, extending the length or breadth of new patents will do little. A new patent, however encompassing, must still compete with existing products. A more promising approach, suggested by the discussion in the previous section, would be to grant new antibiotic patent holders an antitrust exemption that would allow them to exclusively license competing antibiotics, *regardless of the functional group of antibiotic*. With this right, a new patent holder could create a monopoly through merger.

Another approach, recommended by the Infectious Diseases Society of America (IDSA 2004), is to grant a wildcard patent extension to a new antibiotic patent holder. Such an extension would allow the holder to extend for a given number of years the duration of its patent on any one other drug in its portfolio. So, for example, if Pfizer developed a new antibiotic, it would be able to extend its patent on a blockbuster drug such as Lipitor by a number of years. Presumably, this extension would give Pfizer the incentive to invest in antibiotic research an amount up to the additional profit the company might anticipate from extended sales of Lipitor without generic competition.[29] Such a wildcard extension was included in an early version of the Bioshield II bill (S. 975) proposed by Senators Joseph Lieberman and Orrin Hatch in April 2005. That extension would have granted any company that developed a countermeasure to a biological weapon a two-year extension on a patent over any other drug in its portfolio (Divis 2005). If the company had no blockbuster drugs in its portfolio, it could sell its wildcard extension to any other company. This would give every company an incentive to develop a new antibiotic that is as great as the value of the wildcard to, for example, Pfizer, since any company could sell its extension to Pfizer.

The cost of either approach—an antitrust exemption or a wildcard extension—is that using monopoly profits to induce innovation has a high cost in terms of deadweight loss on consumers. Because monopolists price above marginal cost (and even above average cost), individual consumers are denied consumption when the drug's actual cost is less than their willingness to pay. This lost opportunity is the loss of economic efficiency or deadweight loss. The more elastic consumer demand is for antibiotics (with the antitrust exemption) or for a company's blockbuster drug (with the wildcard patent extension), the greater the loss. In political markets, a proxy for this loss—at least in the case of a wildcard patent extension—is opposition from generic

---

29  An important concern with the wildcard extension, especially if it is tradable, is that it may give too much incentive for innovation. The investment in innovation would be as large as the additional rents from the extension, an amount that could run into many billions of dollars in the case of tradable extensions. Although antibiotic resistance has serious human costs, the current and anticipated loss in life may not be worth such a large investment. To put it another way, the investment may be better spent on other health concerns, such as heart disease or HIV. Since resources are limited, allocation of resources to combat resistant bacteria on the margin takes away from resources that could be allocated to other ailments.

drug companies. Not surprisingly, they were vocal in their opposition to Bioshield II. At first they obtained a bar on the sale of the wildcard extension (actually a bar to the acquisition of a company with a wildcard extension) (Divis 2005). They later quashed even the nontradable wildcard extension proposal altogether when the Lieberman-Hatch bill was replaced by an otherwise identical bill (originally S. 1873, S. 2564 as reintroduced on April 9, 2006) from Senator Richard Burr that omitted the wildcard extension (*FDA Week* 2005; Phillips 2005).

## :: GOVERNMENT REWARDS

An alternative to using the carrot of monopoly profits to induce innovation is to employ government research subsidies, tax breaks, or prizes.[30] The argument for this approach is not that it avoids monopoly pricing of a new antibiotic,[31] but rather that it works when there are no monopoly profits to be extracted with a new antibiotic patent. This might be the case when one also employs demand-side strategies to control antibiotic use. In other words, if one wants to curb antibiotic use and at the same time spur innovation, subsidies,

> Either NIH or FDA could assume the job of administering rewards for developing new antibiotics. NIH already judges scientific merit, but it currently does this for noncommercial products and early in the development pipeline.

tax breaks, and prizes are the solution. Antitrust exemptions and wildcard patents might also spur innovation in these circumstances, but they do so at the cost of monopoly pricing outside the scope of the antibiotic that is patented.[32]

Research subsidies would presumably be allocated through the National Institutes of Health (NIH). Tax breaks—specifically, a tax credit for expenditures on research on antibiotics—would be administered by IRS. Either NIH or FDA could assume the job of administering rewards for developing new antibiotics. NIH already judges scientific merit, but it currently does this for noncommercial products and early in the development pipeline. FDA is better situated to conduct *ex post* evaluations of drugs but does not have the capacity to hand out large sums of money.[33]

---

30  For general reviews comparing rewards rather than monopoly rights to encourage innovation, see Shavell and Ypersele (2001) and Abramowicz (2003).

31  Kremer (1998) has proposed a novel alternative to the traditional patent system that addresses the problem of monopoly pricing. Under his patent buyout scheme, the government would award patents to investors and then auction off the patent to the highest bidder. The purpose of the auction is to induce an accurate private valuation of the profit stream that a patent is worth. For most patents, the government would match the highest bidder's price and sell the patented technology at marginal cost. For the remainder, the government would sell the patent to the private winner of the auction. (The purpose is to induce bidders to take the auction seriously.) There are two difficulties with applying this scheme to antibiotics. First, it solves only the monopoly pricing problem. It does not solve the incentive problem where there are competing antibiotics and thus meager profits from the patent. Second, the subset of patents that are actually sold to the highest private bidders has to be random. If it were predictable, then bidders would not take seriously auctions for patents the government ultimately intended to purchase. If the government intended to purchase all antibiotic patents, then it would not be able to value those patents accurately and thus induce optimal investment in the research behind them.

32  Of course, one must balance the deadweight loss from monopoly pricing under an antitrust exemption or patents with the inefficiencies from taxation, which is necessary to fund any research subsidy or prize.

33  More recently, Glennerster and Kremer (2000) proposed "purchase precommitments" to spur innovation. Specifically, the government would commit to purchasing a fixed (large) quantity of a product at a fixed price to induce the development of that product. This concept is very similar to an award except that the government would reduce the monopoly pricing costs of an award by reselling the units it purchased at marginal cost. Therefore,

One drawback to a subsidy, as opposed to an award, is that the government must identify the recipient company before it develops a new antibiotic and risk the possibility that the effort fails. If the government is not very good at picking winners, the cost may be large. An award, however, must be larger than a subsidy to induce any given level of investment because the award requires competing companies to bear the risk of failure. Ordinarily, one might assume that the government is quite good at bearing risk. But in this case the loss is not a financial one borne by all taxpayers—as in the case of the Federal Deposit Insurance Corporation or the Pension Benefit Guaranty Corporation—but a lost health opportunity borne by patients with resistant bacterial infections. Because patients are not particularly suited to bearing this risk, it may be that a large award is warranted. Tax breaks can be structured to behave like a subsidy (e.g., a tax credit for all research expenses) or like an award (e.g., a credit for a clinical trial or marketing expenses). Hence, the choice between subsidies or an award and tax breaks will depend on the structure of the tax break.[34]

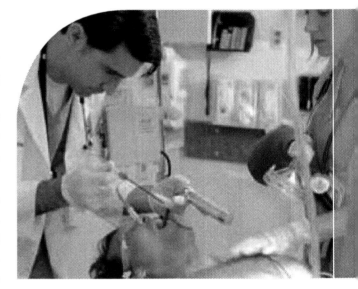

another way to view the purchase commitment is either as an award that requires the winning firm to release its product to the public domain or as an award coupled with a purchase subsidy (Lichtman 1997).

34  An interesting but unexplored option is a variant of an award that has some of the reduced-risk properties of a subsidy: a minimum-return guarantee. Such a policy would give developers of a new antibiotic not an unconditional award but a payment if and only if the return on investment in the new antibiotic failed to reach competitive levels. If the returns did, then no payment would be made. (If each new antibiotic is guaranteed this competitive return, only the costs of developing that specific antibiotic may be used to calculate a competitive return for the antibiotic. If each new functional group of antibiotic is guaranteed a competitive return, then only the costs of research on all new antibiotics should be used to calculate a competitive return. No cross-subsidization of failed nonantibiotic drugs is necessary to encourage investment in antibiotics.) One unique advantage of this minimum-return guarantee is that taxpayers pay not for the full value of a new antibiotic, but only to the extent of the market's failure to properly value that antibiotic. One problem with the scheme, however, is that it may be difficult to calculate the return that a drug company obtains from a new antibiotic. This is related to the problem with rate regulation of public utilities, such as telephone companies. Regulated companies had an incentive to exaggerate their costs to raise rates. Drug companies would have the same incentive to trigger the minimum-return guarantee.

## :: MARKETING

So far this chapter has focused on the development of a new antibiotic. But generating profit from innovation requires not just research but also marketing. The main requirement for marketing is FDA approval. FDA requires that a new drug be both safe and effective (relative to a placebo). This requires three phases of trials. The cost of trials has been estimated to be roughly $125 million per drug (DiMasi, Hansen et al. 2003). Taking into account the time value of money and other indirect expenses, the overall costs of drug approval have been estimated to be as high as $231 million (Ward 1992).[35] These costs may be a significant hurdle to the marketing of a new antibiotic, and thus to its development. One solution may be to lower the requirement for approval of a drug or to speed approval of new drugs. The latter tactic was implemented

35  If one takes into account the cross-subsidization of drugs that fail to get approval, the cost may be as high as $800 million (Powers 2004). In addition, Rubin (2004–2005) suggests that FDA appears (perhaps inadvertently) to have a lower standard for withdrawing approval for antibiotics because of adverse events.

in the Prescription Drug User Fee Acts of 1997 and 2002.[36] These acts required FDA to speed up its process of reviewing drugs and taxed drug applicants to finance the quicker review. The result was a reduction in the time required for review by 3 to 7 percent per year (Berndt, Gottschalk et al. 2006). Critics were concerned that the rapid review came at the cost of safety. Philipson, Berndt et al. (2005) examined this question and estimated that the net effect was a gain for consumers: faster approval saved 180,000 to 310,000 life-years whereas lower implicit safety standards cost at most 56,000 life-years. More importantly for our purposes, the authors estimated that the Prescription Drug User Fee Acts raised the private returns of producers, and thus incentives for innovation, by $11 billion to $13 billion. Although a similar strategy might be recommended for antibiotics, it is unclear whether review times could be significantly reduced beyond levels achieved by the legislation, which already applies to antibiotics.

Another solution could be tax breaks for the cost of obtaining FDA approval. A precedent is the Orphan Drug Act, which, in addition to granting seven years of marketing exclusivity for developers of drugs for rare ailments, also grants developers a credit toward taxes owed equal to 50 percent of clinical testing costs (26 U.S.C. §44(H)). Companies could petition FDA to classify new antibiotics as orphan drugs because, given the practice of reserving new antibiotics for patients with multidrug-resistant infections, fewer than 200,000 persons have a condition for which the drug would be employed. Alternatively, Congress could explicitly extend the act to cover all new antibiotics or adopt an analogous act exclusively for antibiotics. (The Infectious Diseases Society of America has already proposed legislative language toward this end as a modification to the Burr bill.) Depending on the level of innovation desired, Congress could raise the level of the tax credit for clinical testing costs. Research by Lichtenberg and Waldfogel (2003) suggests that the Orphan Drug Act has been relatively successful.[37] The percentage of individuals dying young from rare illnesses fell 6 percent between 1979 and 1998. During the same period, the percentage dying young from more common diseases fell only 2 percent. Thus the act may be credited with a 4 percent reduction in rare disease mortality.[38]

---

37  For a less optimistic view, see Rohde (2000).

38  Space constraints preclude discussion of all policy options for improving the supply of antibiotics, including some creative tactics. For example, because investment in the development of new antibiotics is discouraged by doctors' practice of preferring cheap generics and reserving new antibiotics, an intuitive approach would be formulary controls that do the opposite—reserve generic antibiotics. This would artificially generate demand for and thus investment in new antibiotics. There are downsides that make this option unrealistic. First, costs to patients will rise. These costs are unlikely to be proportional to the resistance externalities that individual use of antibiotics generates. Conventional economic thought holds that incentives to discourage externalities should be proportional to the externality so as not to discourage net beneficial activity. Second, reserving generics will trigger strong opposition from generics manufacturers. In part, this will reflect the first downside. But almost as importantly, it makes this option less politically feasible.

Another approach would be to develop or subsidize diagnostic tests that identify resistant infections. Such tests would make it easier to identify subjects for clinical trials of new antibiotics and thus reduce the costs of obtaining marketing approval from FDA. A risk, however, is that diagnostic tests will also limit use of antibiotics once approved. Doctors may use the tests to avoid giving new antibiotics to patients without resistant infections. This will reduce the returns from developing new antibiotics.

---

36  A related idea, based on a proposal by Grabowski (2003), is to allow companies to get wildcard review priority from FDA in return for developing new antibiotics. The average time taken by FDA to review a nonpriority drug is 18 months; the average time for a priority drug is just 6 months. Grabowski, Vernon et al. (2002) estimate that the value of this incentive is approximately $100 million to $300 million.

## CONCLUSION

The purpose of this chapter was to review the theoretical costs and benefits of the different policy options to encourage pharmaceutical companies to better ration of existing antibiotics and develop new antibiotics. A fundamental question that needs to be addressed in order to move forward with any particular policy, however, is to what extent each policy will actually encourage rationing or promote development. Because no answer is currently available, this chapter closes with three basic research priorities:

1. To what extent will expanding the length and breadth of property rights (directly by the government or via collusive private contracts) encourage drug companies to reduce antibiotic sales?

2. Which policy(ies) would have the greatest impact on encouraging the development of new antibiotics?

3. What level of investment in research is required to discover a new antibiotic, especially one that uses a novel mechanism of action?

# References

Abramowicz, M. B. (2003). "Perfecting Patent Prizes." *Vanderbilt Law Review* 56: 114–236.

Albus, A., E. Pesci, et al. (1997). "Vfr Controls Quorum Sensing in *Pseudomonas aeruginosa*." *Journal of Bacteriology* 179(12): 3928–35.

Bartlett, J. G., P. G. Auwaerter, et al. (eds.). (2007). "Johns Hopkins Division of Infectious Diseases Antibiotic Guide." http://hopkins-abxguide.org/terminals/antibiotics_navigator.cfm?id=1&p=1 (accessed January 19, 2007).

BCC Research. (2001). "Antibiotics Market Expected to Cross $34.5 Billion by 2006." Press release, Dec. 12. www.bccresearch.com/editors/RB-155.html (accessed May 31, 2006).

Berndt, E. R., A. H. B. Gottschalk, et al. (2006). "Assessing the Impacts of the Prescription Drug User Fee Acts (PDUFA) on the FDA Approval Process." Forum for Health Economics & Policy, *Forum: Frontiers in Health Policy Research* 8(2). http://www.bepress.com/fhep/8/2 (accessed May 31, 2006).

Bosso, J. A. (2005). "The Antimicrobial Armamentarium: Evaluating Current and Future Treatment Options." *Pharmacotherapy* 25(10): 55S–62S.

Braun, J. (2006). "Trial Phage." *Seed.* Feb/Mar.

Brown, S. P. A., and W. C. Gruben. (1997). "Intellectual Property Rights and Product Effectiveness." *Economic Review*, Federal Reserve Bank of Dallas 1997(4): 15–20.

Bull, J. J., B. R. Levin, et al. (2002). "Dynamics of Success and Failure in Phage and Antibiotic Therapy in Experimental Infections." *BMC Microbiology* 2: 35.

Bush, K. (2004). "Antibacterial Drug Discovery in the 21st Century." *Clinical Microbiology & Infection* 10(Suppl. 4): 10–17.

Campbell, A. (2003). "The Future of Bacteriophage Biology." *Nature Reviews. Genetics* 4(6): 471–77.

Coase, R. H. (1960). "The Problem of Social Cost." *Journal of Law and Economics* 3: 1–44.

Coase, R. (1972). "Durable Goods Monopolists." *Journal of Law and Economics* 15: 143–50.

Cromie, W. J. (2001). "Resistance to Antibiotics is Reversed." *Harvard Gazette*, Sept. 20. http//www.news.harvard.edu/gazette/2001/09.20/18-antibiotics.html (accessed May 31, 2006).

DiMasi, J., R. Hansen, et al. (2003). "The Price of Innovation: New Estimates of Drug Development Costs." *Journal of Health Economics* 22: 151–85.

Divis, D. A. (2005). "BioWar: Bioshield Wild-Card Patent Curbed." *Washington Times.* http://www.washtimes.com/upi-breaking/20050427-091025-5443r.htm (accessed May 31, 2006).

Ellickson, R. (1986). "Of Coase and Cattle: Dispute Resolution Among Neighbors in Shasta County." *Stanford Law Review* 38: 623–87.

Ellison, S. F., and J. K. Hellerstein. (1999). The Economics of Antibiotics: An Exploratory Study. *Measuring the Prices of Medical Treatments.* J. E. Triplett (ed.) Washington, DC: Brookings Institution Press, 118–151.

Epstein, R. A. (2002). "The Dubious Constitutionality of the Copyright Term Extension Act." *Loyola of Los Angeles Law Review* 36: 123–58.

*Evans v. Jordan.* 8 F. Cas. 873. (1813).

FDA. (2004). "Challenge and Opportunity on the Critical Path to New Medical Products." http://www.fda.gov/oc/initiatives/critical path/whitepaper.html (accessed May 31, 2006). Food and Drug Administration.

*FDA Week.* (2005). "Burr's Bioshield II Bill Does Not Include Wildcard Exclusivity." *Inside Washington's FDA Week* 11(42).

Fidler, D. P. (1998). "Legal Issues Associated with Antimicrobial Drug Resistance." *Emerging Infectious Diseases* 4(2): 169–77.

Forslid, R. (2006). "Can We Trust Monopolistic Firms as Suppliers of Vaccines for the Avian Influenza?" Working paper 2005:2. Stockholm, Sweden: Stockholm University.

Fuqua, W. C., S. C. Winans, et al. (1994). "Quorum Sensing in Bacteria: The LuxR-LuxI Family of Cell Density-Responsive Transcriptional Regulators." *Journal of Bacteriology* 176(2): 269–75.

Gilcrest, L. (2004). "U.S. Seeks to Boost Drug Innovation with New Incentives." Nov. 8. http://www.investors.com/breakingnews.asp?journal id=23889518&brk=1 (accessed May 31, 2006).

Glennerster, R., and M. Kremer. (2000). "A Better Way to Spur Medical Research and Development." *Regulation* 23(2): 34-39.

Gordon, H. S. (1954). "The Economic Theory of a Common-Property Resource: The Fishery." *Journal of Political Economy* 62(2): 124–42.

Grabowski, H. (2003). "Increasing R&D Incentives for Neglected Diseases—Lessons from the Orphan Drug Act." Working paper 03-13. Durham, NC: Duke University.

Grabowski, H., J. Vernon, et al. (2002). "Returns on Research and Development for the 1990s: New Drug Introductions." *PharmacoEconomics* 20(S3): 11–29.

Gray, L. (2004). "Pandemic Control: Resistant Organisms and Emerging Threats." BCC Research Report PHM042A. Norwalk, CT: BCC Research.

Hardin, G. (1968). "The Tragedy of the Commons." *Science* 162: 1243–48.

Harrison, P. F. and J. Lederberg (eds.). (1998). *Antimicrobial Resistance: Issues and Options, Workshop Report.* Forum on Emerging Infections. Washington, DC: Institute of Medicine.

Hotelling, H. (1931). "The Economics of Exhaustible Resources." *Journal of Political Economy* 39(2): 137–75.

IDSA. (2004). "Bad Bugs, No Drugs: As Antibiotic Discovery Stagnates ... A Public Health Crisis Brews." http://www.idsociety.org/pa/IDSA_Paper4_final_web.pdf (accessed May 31, 2006). Infectious Diseases Society of America.

Kades, E. (2005). "Preserving a Precious Resource: Rationalizing the Use of Antibiotics." *Northwestern University Law Review* 99: 611–74.

Kim, J., and J. Mahoney. (2005). "Property Rights Theory, Transaction Costs Theory, and Agency Theory: An Organizational Economics Approach to Strategic Management." *Managerial & Decision Economics* 26: 223–42.

Kitch, E. W. (1977). "The Nature and Function of the Patent System." *Journal of Law and Economics* 20(2): 265–90.

Kremer, M. (1998). "Patent Buyouts: A Mechanism for Encouraging Innovation." *Quarterly Journal of Economics* 113: 1137–67.

Kremer, M., and C. M. Snyder. (2004). "Why Is There No AIDS Vaccine?" Working Paper No. 111. Cambridge, MA: Center for International Development at Harvard University.

Laxminarayan, R. (2001). "Fighting Antibiotic Resistance: Can Economic Incentives Play a Role?" *Resources,* Resources for the Future 143: 9–12.

Levin, B. R., and J. J. Bull. (2004). "Population and Evolutionary Dynamics of Phage Therapy." *Nature Reviews. Microbiology* 2(2): 166–73.

Lichtenberg, F. R., and J. Waldfogel. (2003). "Does Misery Love Company? Evidence from Pharmaceutical Markets Before and After the Orphan Drug Act." Working paper 9750. Cambridge, MA: NBER (National Bureau of Economic Research).

Lichtman, D. G. (1997). "Pricing Prozac: Why the Government Should Subsidize the Purchase of Patented Pharmaceuticals." *Harvard Journal of Law & Technology* 11: 123–39.

Martin, R. (2003). "How Ravenous Soviet Viruses Will Save the World." *Wired.* 11.10.

Nachbar, T. B. (2004). "Intellectual Property and Constitutional Norms." *Columbia Law Review* 104: 272–362.

Philipson, T., E. Berndt, et al. (2005). "Assessing the Safety and Efficacy of the FDA: The Case of the Prescription Drug User Fee Acts." Working paper 11724. Cambridge, MA: NBER (National Bureau of Economic Research).

Philipson, T., S. Mechoulan, et al. (2006). "IP & External Consumption Effects: Generalizations from Health Care Markets." Working paper 11930. Cambridge, MA: NBER (National Bureau of Economic Research).

Phillips, Z. (2005). "In 2005, Vaccine Makers Got Their Wish: Liability Protection." CQ Homeland Security, Dec. 30. www.cq.com (accessed May 31, 2006).

Powers, J. H. (2004). "Antimicrobial Drug Development—The Past, the Present, and the Future." *Clinical Microbiology & Infection* 10 (Suppl. 4): 23–31.

Radetsky, P. (1996). "The Good Virus." Discover 17(11).

Rasmussen, T. B. and M. Givskov. (2006). "Quorum Sensing Inhibitors: A Bargain of Effects." *Microbiology* 152(4): 895–904.

Rohde, D. D. (2000). "The Orphan Drug Act: An Engine of Innovation? At What Cost?" *Food and Drug Law Journal* 55: 125–43.

Rubin, P. H. (2004–2005). "The FDA's Antibiotic Resistance." *Regulation* (Winter): 34–37

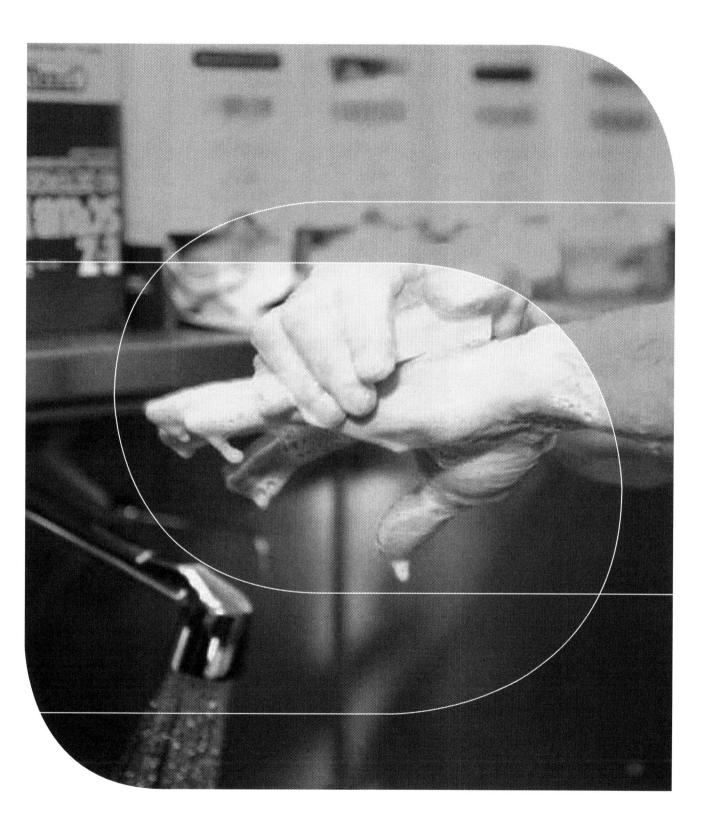

Schoolnik, G. K., W. C. Summers, et al. (2004). "Phage Offer a Real Alternative." *Nature Biotechnology* 22(5): 505–506; author reply 506–507.

*Science.* (1994). "Funding Crunch Hobbles Antibiotic Resistance Research." 264 (April 15): 362.

Service, R. F. (2004). "Orphan Drugs of the Future." *Science* 303 (Mar. 19): 1798.

Shavell, S., and T. V. Ypersele. (2001). "Rewards Versus Intellectual Property Rights." *Journal of Law and Economics* 44: 525–47.

Spellberg, B., J. H. Powers, et al. (2004). "Trends in Antimicrobial Drug Development: Implications for the Future." *Clinical Infectious Diseases* 38: 1279–86.

Stinson, S.C. 1996. "Drug Firms Restock Antibacterial Arsenal." *Chemical & Engineering News* (Sept. 23): 75–100.

Sulakvelidze, A. (2006). Personal communication with Elliot Klein, Resources for the Future. March 28, 2006.

Talbot, G. H., J. Bradley, et al. (2006). "Bad Bugs Need Drugs: An Update on the Development Pipeline from Antimicrobial Availability Task Force of the Infectious Diseases Society of America." *Clinical Infectious Diseases* 42: 657–68.

Tanouye, E. (1996). "Drug Makers Go All Out to Squash 'Superbugs.'" *Wall Street Journal*, June 25, B1, B9.

Travis, J. (1994). "Reviving the Antibiotic Miracle?" *Science* 264(April 15): 360–62.

Tufts Center for Drug Development. (2001). "Tufts Center for the Study of Drug Development Pegs Cost of a New Prescription Medicine at $802 Million." http://csdd.tufts.edu/NewsEvents/RecentNews.asp?newsid=6 (accessed May 31, 2006).

*U.S. v. Socony-Vacuum Oil Co.* 310 U.S. 150. (1940).

Ward, M. (1992). "Drug Approval Overregulation." *Regulation* 15(4): 47–53.

Westwater, C., L. M. Kasman, et al. (2003). "Use of Genetically Engineered Phage to Deliver Antimicrobial Agents to Bacteria: An Alternative Therapy for Treatment of Bacterial Infections." *Antimicrobial Agents and Chemotherapy* 47(4): 1301–307.

Williams, P. (2006). "Quorum Sensing in Human Pathogens." *International Journal of Medical Microbiology* 296(2-3): 57–59.

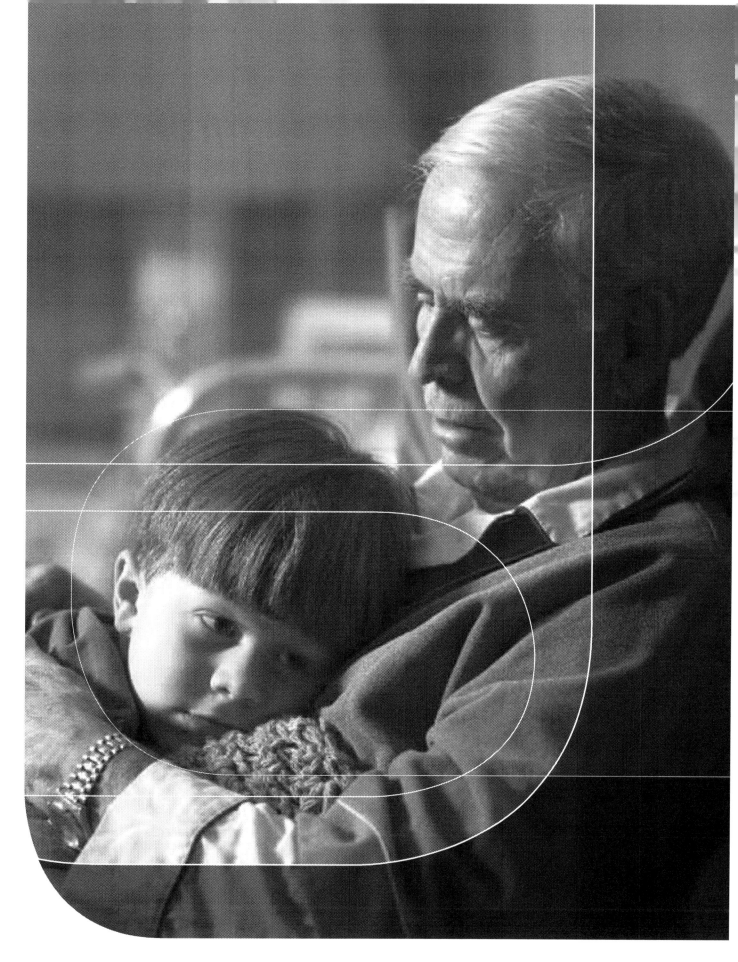

# 8

# Next **Steps**

*Ramanan Laxminarayan*

*When you want to cook a frog, they say, don't throw it into boiling water—it will only jump out.*
*Instead, place the frog in tepid water and, ever so slowly, increase the heat.*

Much like the frog that is unaware that it is being cooked, our reaction to the antibiotic resistance problem has been to wait for a crisis before responding—but the frequency of resistance has been increasing slowly and steadily. When resistance reaches crisis levels, it may be too late. Meanwhile, thousands of people continue to die or suffer from a cause that does not show up on any death certificate. A crisis need not be a sudden, uncontrollable outbreak of a resistant pathogen. Many believe that the emergence and spread of deadly infections like community-acquired MRSA already constitutes a crisis. Perhaps we will see drug-resistant pneumonia and MRSA in large numbers of patients afflicted with avian influenza, or perhaps the prevalence of *Clostridium difficile*, which by itself is not a drug-resistant pathogen but whose survival and proliferation have been facilitated by widespread antibiotic use, will reach epidemic proportions. Many deaths during the influenza epidemic of 1918 are thought to have been caused by untreatable bacterial infections—bacterial pneumonia, and not just pneumonia caused by streptococci but also staphylococcus-associated pneumonia. The combination of today's highly virulent MRSA with an outbreak of avian flu could have devastating consequences.

It is perplexing why so little attention is paid to finding solutions to the antibiotic resistance problem when it has such catastrophic potential. One is reminded of the years of neglect that led to the failure of the levees and the destruction of New Orleans during Hurricane Katrina. Even if policymakers are not motivated to act in preparation for such a medical eventuality, a more immediate concern—the increasing costs of health care and the consequent difficulty of bringing large numbers of uninsured people under the umbrella of pooled-risk financing—may spur action.

Regardless of when policy action is forthcoming, policymakers will need a playbook of carefully considered ideas. Our objective in writing this report has been to sketch the outlines of such a playbook, notwithstanding that more basic science and policy research may be needed on some of the ideas. A summary of policy actions, their pros and cons, and the actors involved is presented in Table 8.1.

This report has outlined a plan to change incentives to address antibiotic resistance in health care, not just in the immediate term (such as by changing Medicare reimbursement rules, subsidizing hospital infection control and diagnostics, or imposing stricter state standards for reporting hospital infections) but also in the longer term, to ensure a sustainable and affordable supply of antibiotics into the foreseeable future. After all, new drugs take at least 10 to 15 years to develop, and policies changing how antibiotics are used will take years to be implemented and have an effect on resistance.

■

## Main messages

Our main conclusion is that antibiotic resistance is an important and growing challenge to health and health care systems. It raises the cost and lowers the effectiveness of health care in the United States and will have potentially serious consequences if not addressed now. Although the underlying causes appear to be, broadly speaking, overuse of antibiotics and inadequate hospital infection control, the deeper reasons relate to incentives. A policy solution will have to address incentives that affect how individuals, physicians, institutions, and pharmaceutical companies demand, use, and produce antibiotics. The changes in the behavior of humans must, in turn, effectively change the microbial world. These issues are not unique to antibiotics, however. Managing incentives is a challenge with the use of any resource, whether oil or fish, and the lessons learned in those contexts can be valuable here.

We have critically and objectively evaluated various policy options to address antibiotic resistance, and on the basis of this evaluation, we make five general observations about the policy solutions.

1. Policy solutions tend to focus either on changing incentives for how individual actors deal with antibiotic use or infection control (by changing how hospitals get reimbursed for hospital acquired infections, for instance), or on exercising federal or state government oversight (by requiring reporting of hospital infections, for instance). This report identifies the incentive problems associated with the latter type of regulatory policy and generally finds greater support for the former, the incentive-altering policies. Government action is needed but is more likely to be effective when focused on changing incentives (say, for new drug development) than on just mandating standards.

2. Much of the public debate on dealing with antibiotic resistance has dealt with lowering antibiotic use. There is a need to broaden the discussion of policy alternatives beyond simply educating health care providers to reduce antibiotic use. We know that antibiotic use leads to resistance, but it is unclear to what extent education alone can lower antibiotic use and how much this will slow resistance. Dealing with resistance will require careful rethinking and restructuring of the incentives for infection control within hospitals and vaccination policies in the community.

Lowering antibiotic use involves a tension between what is good for the individual patient—important from the prescriber's perspective—and what is good for the rest of society. Resolving this tension between sound medicine and sound public health is one feature of the problem; preventing the spread of infections and using a diversity of antibiotics, in contrast, are policy options that do not require balancing the individual and the public good.

3. Our policy goal should go beyond minimizing resistance, since that may be best achieved by not using antibiotics at all. Antibiotics serve a useful social purpose, but we have to balance the benefits of their use to individuals and to the rest of society (by lowering the chance that one patient's infection will spread to others) against the costs that are largely borne by society in the form of lower future effectiveness.

4. Successful policy solutions should incorporate an understanding of ecology and evolutionary biology. A sustainable antibiotics policy must recognize that drug resistance and new drug development are two facets of the ongoing process of coevolution between humans and microbes. New drugs can provide a temporary solution only until microbes catch up through the process of evolution. Moreover, new targets for antibiotics may be increasingly difficult to find, and there may be cross-resistance between old and new antibiotics. Antibiotic efficacy is a renewable resource, but only on very long time scales. Meanwhile, policy must focus on extending the useful therapeutic life of existing drugs, and this requires a change in human behavior that leads to change in microbial communities. To be effective, policy must consider population biology and microbial community ecology, and this will require new basic research, including research to identify microbial interactions that can be exploited to manage resistance.

5. We need to integrate our thinking of supply-side and demand-side policy objectives. Efforts to protect new antibiotics from drug resistance by keeping them on the sidelines potentially reduce incentives for new drug development by the pharmaceutical industry. Similarly, having a supply of new antibiotics that are fundamentally different from existing drugs expands our options by lowering selection pressure for resistance to evolve to existing drugs. Solutions that focus only on the supply side or only on the demand side may be less effective in the long term than solutions that are mindful of the interrelatedness between how we use existing antibiotics and incentives to produce new antibiotics.

Empirical research can inform our current understanding of which policy solutions are most likely to improve sustainable antibiotic use. Much of the discussion of ways to change incentives for patients, physicians, and other agents to behave optimally with respect to resistance is based on a theoretical understanding of economics and the law. However, there are knowledge gaps that prevent progression to an implementation stage.

■
___

## Future policy research and dialogue

This report provides an objective evaluation of various policy alternatives, but the assessment is challenged by important gaps in our understanding of these alternatives. Our call for more data and research is not just a nod to the established norm; our goal is to provide the biological, medical, and economic analysis that can directly inform policy decisions. Although we have evaluated incentives and motivating factors from a theoretical perspective, policymakers will undoubtedly need stronger evidence to act on such policies as subsidizing infection control in hospitals. Policy research is needed to empirically test, using pilot studies and model-based approaches, the effects of some of the more immediate solutions related to changing prescribing behavior and hospital infection control. Policy pilots will be important for determining the impact of greater cost-sharing for antibiotic prescriptions and patient outcomes, and for calculating the effect of subsidizing substitutes for antibiotics that relieve symptoms, thereby reducing antibiotic use. These studies will be useful in understanding what proportion of antibiotic use can be avoided without harming patient outcomes. Modeling will have to be used for other approaches, such as the overall economic impact of antibiotic use and better reporting of resistance levels in hospitals. A natural outcome of this research will be prioritizing policy changes and identifying those most likely to have a significant impact on resistance.

Going forward, it is important not just to engage in policy research but also to reconcile diverse viewpoints among the broad range of stakeholders, ranging from consumer groups and physicians to pharmaceutical companies and health insurers. All of these stakeholders are committed to a long-term future for antibiotics: after all, no one is better off with drugs that do not work. However, specific policy proposals may be more or less palatable to different groups, and it will therefore be important to engage multiple stakeholder groups, such as the Interagency Task Force on Antimicrobial Resistance, the Infectious Diseases Society of America, the Academy of Managed Care Pharmacy, the American Hospitals Association, and the Joint Commission on Accreditation of Health care Organizations, in an expanded, multidisciplinary consultation process to develop consensus around policy solutions that will have a significant impact on how we use and develop antibiotics.

## CONCLUSION

At this time, death from a drug-resistant pathogen, although increasing in frequency, is not yet a concern for most Americans. Many infections that are resistant to common antibiotics typically respond to other, more expensive drugs. However, running out of the cheapest antibiotics is somewhat like running out of oil. Just as oil is relatively cheap and convenient but not our only energy source, so generic antibiotics are inexpensive and available but may not be the only way to treat infectious diseases. Losing drugs that cost pennies a dose and moving to more expensive antibiotics, the newest of which can cost thousands of dollars, can have a profound impact on the health care system as a whole and especially on the poor and uninsured, who are most likely to have to pay directly for their care.

Nevertheless, the time may come when even our most powerful antibiotics will fail. The proposals in this report are meant to offer a guide to policy and research to address this crisis now, rather than waiting until the pressure on policymakers to act —even in the absence of information—is unavoidable. The proposals in this report are meant to offer a guide to prepare for and respond to such a crisis, when there will undoubtedly be far greater pressure on policymakers to act. The ultimate goal should be to develop and implement policy solutions that will ensure the sustainability of antibiotic effectiveness for the next hundred years.

| TABLE 8.1 | EXTENDING THE CURE: SUMMARY OF POLICY OPTIONS | | | |
|---|---|---|---|---|
| POLICY | DESCRIPTION | ACTORS | PROS | CONS |
| CONTROLLING ANTIBIOTIC USE IN HOSPITALS AND OUTPATIENT SETTINGS | | | | |
| Increase cost-sharing for prescriptions | • Increase copayments<br>• Restrict prescribing through formularies<br>• Impose delay for fulfillment of some prescriptions for certain infections | • Insurance companies<br>• Pharmacies<br>• State and federal governments | • Patients will use fewer antibiotics | • May not distinguish between "appropriate" and "inappropriate" use |
| Use public information campaigns | • Educate physicians and patients to discourage inappropriate prescribing | • Doctors (professional societies)<br>• Patient and consumer groups<br>• State and federal government | • Is inexpensive and simple to implement | • May not yield sufficiently large or permanent reductions in use |
| Restrict prescribing by physicians | • Require preapproval for some or all antibiotics<br>• Restrict ability of physicians to prescribe antibiotics | • Doctors and hospitals<br>• State and federal governments | • Circumvents current lack of incentives to reduce inappropriate prescribing | • May inhibit patient-physician relationship<br>• May discourage appropriate antibiotic use |
| Change prescribing patterns in hospital and outpatient settings | • Monitor and present feedback of prescribing patterns compared with peers<br>• Use pay-for-performance measures | • Professional medical associations<br>• Hospitals | • Creates incentives, since physicians care about their reputation and performance | • May discourage all antibiotic use unless feedback distinguishes between appropriate and inappropriate use |
| | • Conserve new and powerful antibiotics for cases where first-line drugs do not work | • Professional medical associations<br>• CDC<br>• Hospitals | • Maintains viability of new antibiotics longer | • Increases resistance to first-line drugs<br>• Is inefficient from ecological standpoint because diversity of antibiotics may be helpful<br>• Decreases incentive to develop new antibiotics |
| | • Switch from broad-spectrum to narrow-spectrum antibiotics | • Doctors | • Reduces opportunities for resistance to arise | • Few rapid tests to determine pathogen are available<br>• Doctors have few incentives to use narrow-spectrum drugs<br>• Is difficult to switch from broad- to narrow-spectrum drugs once therapy has begun<br>• Pharmaceutical industry has few incentives to develop narrow-spectrum antibiotics |
| | • Cycle or rotate drugs | • Doctors and hospitals | • Ecological models suggest this may reduce risks of resistance | • Has not yet been validated in limited trials<br>• Could be costly to implement<br>• Resistance may reemerge rapidly when drug is reintroduced<br>• There may not be enough antibiotics for rotation in each case |

CONTINUED ON PAGE 162

| TABLE 8.1 | EXTENDING THE CURE: SUMMARY OF POLICY OPTIONS (CONTINUED) |

| POLICY | DESCRIPTION | ACTORS | PROS | CONS |
|---|---|---|---|---|
| Change prescribing patterns in hospital and outpatient settings (continued) | • Use two or more antibiotics in combination | • Doctors (professional societies) | • Ecological models suggest this may be effective at slowing down evolution of resistance | • Empirical work has not yet validated many combinations<br>• May compound side effects |
| | • Employ antibiotic heterogeneity (concurrent use of multiple antibiotics on different patients) | • Doctors (professional societies) | • Ecological models suggest this may be effective at slowing down evolution of resistance<br>• Heterogeneity may already be at work since not all patients receive same antibiotic | • Multiple antibiotics may not always be available to treat all conditions |
| | • Increase doses while shortening length of therapy | • Doctors | • May reduce risks of resistance | • Still leaves long tail for recrudescence |
| Provide substitutes | • Promote antibiotic substitutes (e.g., cold packs) in cases where antibiotics are not necessary (e.g., flu)<br>• Shift some remedies from prescription to over the counter<br>• Rethink limited access to pseudoephedrine | • Managed-care organizations<br>• Insurance companies<br>• State and federal governments | • Simple, does not require major changes, lets physicians reduce antibiotic use without reducing patient satisfaction | • Substitutes lack effectiveness<br>• Impact on antibiotic use has not been widely studied |
| Impose tax, quota, or permit | • Tax antibiotic use either generally or selectively | • State and federal governments | • Creates strong incentive to reduce use | • Does not differentiate between appropriate and inappropriate use<br>• Insurance shields intended targets from tax burden |
| Improve diagnostic accuracy | • Improve diagnostic tests<br>• Improve decision rules on when to use antibiotics | • Doctors (professional societies)<br>• Hospitals<br>• Medical schools<br>• State and federal governments | • Delays drug therapy until need for antibiotics is certain<br>• Encourages use of narrow-spectrum drugs when appropriate<br>• Decision rules are inexpensive and can easily be incorporated into clinical therapy | • Decision rules lack specificity<br>• Some diagnostic tests are expensive and invasive |
| Research novel ecological approaches | • Test all novel approaches | • NIH<br>• Drug companies | • Many ecological strategies (at both population level and patient level) would use existing antibiotics more effectively | • Who should bear cost of developing these strategies is not clear |
| | • Explore probiotics ("good bacteria") | • Doctors<br>• Drug companies | • Can be used to fill niche left by antibiotic use | • Public health value of probiotics is uncertain and not well studied |
| | • Employ bacteriophages ("bacteria eaters") or other biological control agents | • Drug companies | • Bacteriophages can attack and adapt to resistant bacteria and reduce need for antibiotics | • Approach is largely speculative<br>• Bacteriophages may themselves cause toxicity |
| | • Interfere with bacterial quorum sensing (which facilitates invasion of host) | • Drug companies | • Could prevent bacteria from "attacking" or cause bacteria to "attack" prematurely | • May not work for all bacteria<br>• May have side effects on helpful bacteria<br>• Feasibility is unknown |

| POLICY | DESCRIPTION | ACTORS | PROS | CONS |
|---|---|---|---|---|
| HOSPITAL INFECTION CONTROL | | | | |
| Clear colonizing infections in incoming patients | • Use alternative antibiotic to clear resistant colonized bacteria in patients susceptible to infection | • Doctors (professional societies)<br>• Hospitals | • Reduces the number of antibiotic resistant infections | • Resistance to alternatives may develop |
| Employ surveillance and patient isolation | • Screen all patients on admission (active surveillance) and isolate patients who test positive | • Hospitals | • Reduces likelihood of antibiotic-resistant pathogens entering hospital<br>• Reduces chances of transmission | • Is costly and time consuming<br>• Stigmatizes infected patients<br>• Does not completely eliminate possibility of transmission |
| | • Screen only patients at risk (selective active surveillance): those who were recently hospitalized or had previous resistant infections | • Hospitals | • Reduces likelihood of antibiotic-resistant pathogens entering hospital<br>• Is less costly than screening everyone | • Is costly and time consuming<br>• Requires electronic medical records |
| Reduce transmission by health care workers | • Reduce patient cohorting (number of patients seen by each nurse) | • Hospitals<br>• Health care workers<br>• Doctors | • Could reduce transmission | • Is costly and difficult to implement and enforce |
| | • Improve hygiene through education (on hand washing, gloves, gowns) | • Hospitals | • Could reduce transmission | • May require installation of hand-washing stations<br>• Incentives to follow guidelines are lacking<br>• Long-term impact of interventions is unclear |
| | • Improve hygiene through pay-for-performance measures (such as for achieving certain target rates for hand washing) | • Hospitals | • Could change incentives for health care workers and doctors | • May require installation of hand-washing stations<br>• Effect of changing incentives may wear off |
| Reduce transmission by patients and visitors | • Improve cleaning of visitors' and patients' rooms | • Hospitals | • Removes pathogens, reducing likelihood of transmission<br>• Does not affect clinical practice | • Is expensive but may be cost-effective if carried out in many or all health care institutions |
| Promote regional cooperation | • Enforce regional cooperation and information sharing to improve hospital infection control at regional level | • Hospitals<br>• State and local governments | • Ensures coordinated infection control<br>• Reduces free-riding by individual facilities | • Hospitals may not cooperate<br>• May be difficult and costly to ensure cooperation |
| Require hospital infection and resistance reporting | • Require hospitals to report levels of hospital-acquired infections and resistance | • Hospitals<br>• State and federal governments | • Increases transparency<br>• Creates incentive to reduce levels of infection | • Creates disincentive to monitoring among hospitals with high levels of infection<br>• Creates incentive to cherry-pick patients<br>• May encourage lawsuits by patients with hospital-acquired infections<br>• Is difficult to enforce |

CONTINUED ON PAGE 164

TABLE 8.1

## EXTENDING THE CURE: SUMMARY OF POLICY OPTIONS (CONTINUED)

| POLICY | DESCRIPTION | ACTORS | PROS | CONS |
|---|---|---|---|---|
| Change hospital incentives | • Link hospital reimbursement to levels of infection | • Hospitals<br>• Insurance companies | • Creates incentive to reduce levels of infection to get full reimbursement | • Is difficult to implement<br>• Creates incentive to cherry-pick patients |
| | • Examine legal avenues for responding to resistance | • Lawyers<br>• Hospitals | • Creates incentive to reduce levels of infection to avoid medical malpractice lawsuits | • Creates disincentive to monitor levels of infection<br>• Legal system may be inappropriate and expensive for determining medical causation<br>• Is politically infeasible because of pushback from providers |
| | • Consider impact of infections on hospital budgets and organizational structure | • Hospitals<br>• Medical research institutions<br>• Government agencies | • Multidisciplinary research could identify organizational issues that reduce hospital incentives to conduct surveillance | • Actors are nonspecific<br>• Mandate is unclear |
| | • Include infection control in hospital accreditation and health care quality ratings | • Hospitals<br>• JCAHO<br>• Health care quality organizations (e.g., Leapfrog) | • Coverage would be comprehensive<br>• Quality indicators are increasingly important in health care purchasing decisions | • JCAHO monitors only hospital protocols, not levels of infection<br>• Current process is designed to catch egregious violators of medical practice<br>• Infections are only one consideration in determining quality of health care facility |
| **ROLE OF GOVERNMENT** | | | | |
| Incentives to encourage development of new antibiotics | • Fund basic scientific research to identify new organisms | • NIH | • Reduces cost of creating new antibiotics | • Introduces issues of patent ownership and royalties |
| | • Speed up approval of antibiotics | • FDA | • Reduces cost and increases return from creating new antibiotics | • Safety may be traded off for speed |
| | • Increase financial incentives for companies developing new antibiotics | • Congress | • Increases incentive for pharmaceutical companies to create new antibiotics | • Is costly<br>• Does not solve the common property problem (many firms exploiting the same pool of effectiveness)<br>• Does not encourage innovation |
| | • Tie financial incentives for companies to efficacy of drug | • Congress | • Gives pharmaceutical companies incentive to maintain efficacy of their drugs | • Appropriate standards for efficacy must be developed<br>• Is costly |
| | • Create new agency to fund research | • Congress<br>• Proposed Biomedical Advanced Research and Development Agency<br>• Other government agency | • Lowers cost of creating new antibiotics<br>• Could solve common property and innovation problems through oversight | • Government may not be best positioned to pick winners<br>• Is costly |

| POLICY | DESCRIPTION | ACTORS | PROS | CONS |
|---|---|---|---|---|
| **Make federal government steward of antibiotic effectiveness** | • Create separate agency within FDA to handle antibiotic effectiveness | • FDA<br>• Congress | • Empowers FDA to better control antibiotics<br>• Provides greater financial support for federal antibiotic stewardship | • May require congressional authorization |
| | • Pass comprehensive legislation to protect antibiotic effectiveness | • Congress | • Recognizes vital national interest in effectiveness of antibiotics<br>• Funds programs to help conserve effectiveness of existing drugs and support investments in new drugs<br>• Coordinates actions to manage antibiotic effectiveness and develop new antibiotics | • Congressional action to protect natural resources has mixed track record |
| | • Mandate use of pneumococcal vaccine | • State and federal governments | • Lowers rates of infection and thus use of antibiotics | • Vaccine is currently expensive |
| | • Promote and subsidize best practices to lower hospital infections and resistance | • Medicare<br>• Medicaid | • Makes better use of hospital resources | • Is expensive<br>• Mandate to do this is unclear |
| | • Facilitate innovation by conducting field experiments | • Medicare<br>• Medicaid | • Creates significant societal benefits through large-scale experiments to slow evolution of resistance | • Is expensive<br>• Mandate to do this is unclear |
| | • Require broad infection control programs as condition of participation | • Medicare<br>• Medicaid | • Benefits all patients | • May deny coverage to segment of population |
| | • Require specific techniques to qualify | • Medicare<br>• Medicaid | • Improves care for all patients<br>• Establishes standard of care for medical malpractice suits | • May deny coverage to segment of population |
| | • Create codes (hospitals' diagnosis-related group and physicians' common procedure terminology) to track resistant infections and prescribing patterns | • Medicare<br>• Medicaid | • Creates transparency<br>• Provides more data on problem | • Is difficult to change codes<br>• Hospitals may engage in "creative" coding |

CONTINUED ON PAGE 166

**TABLE 8.1**

**EXTENDING THE CURE: SUMMARY OF POLICY OPTIONS** (CONTINUED)

| POLICY | DESCRIPTION | ACTORS | PROS | CONS |
|---|---|---|---|---|
| Change patent and antitrust laws to alter incentives for pharmaceutical companies to conserve anitbiotic effectiveness | • Allow infinite patents for antibiotics | • Congress | • Increases incentives to develop antibiotics and maintain their efficacy | • Patent law is intended to encourage innovation, not solve commons problem |
| | • Define patent law for antibiotics over functional resistance groups | • Congress | • Reduces likelihood of resistance arising to classes of drugs under competing patents<br>• Increases incentive to maintain efficacy of antibiotics | • Reduces incentives for companies to create new antibiotics in functional resistance groups they don't own |
| | • Grant *sui generis* rights over antibiotics | • Congress | • Reduces number of competing drugs in same functional group | • Creates issue of ownership of rights<br>• Generic drug makers may protest |
| | • Relax antitrust law | • Congress | • Allows patenting of functional resistance groups | • Is politically difficult<br>• Loss of efficiency may be great |
| | • Harmonize property rights and antitrust laws across countries | • International treaty organizations (such as WTO) | • Transcends national boundaries for this international problem | • Other countries cannot be forced to comply |
| | • Create wildcard patent extension (for developer of antibiotic to use on existing patent or sell to another company) | • Congress | • Increases incentive to develop new antibiotics | • Is costly<br>• May raise objections from other drug makers |

CDC = Centers for Disease Control

FDA = Food and Drug Administration

NIH = National Institutes of Health

JCAHO = Joint Commission on Accreditation of Health care Organizations

WTO = World Trade Organization

# Acronyms and Abbreviations

**ARI:** antibiotic-resistant infection

**BARDA:** Biomedical Advanced Research and Development Agency

**Bt:** *Bacillus thuringiensis*

**CA-MRSA:** community-acquired methicillin-resistant *Staphylococcus aureus*

**CDC:** Centers for Disease Control and Prevention

**CMS:** Centers for Medicare and Medicaid Services

**COBRA:** Consolidated Omnibus Budget Reconciliation Act

**CPT:** common procedure terminology

**DRG:** diagnosis-related group

**EARSS:** European Antimicrobial Resistance Surveillance System

**EPA:** U.S. Environmental Protection Agency

**FDA:** U.S. Food and Drug Administration

**FRG:** functional resistance group

**HA-MRSA:** hospital-acquired methicillin-resistant *Staphylococcus aureus*

**HAI:** hospital-acquired infection

**HHI:** Herfindahl-Hirschman Index

**HHS:** U.S. Department of Health and Human Services

**HIC:** hospital infection control

**HICPAC:** Hospital Infection Control Practices Advisory Committee

**HMO:** health maintenance organization

**IDSA:** Infectious Diseases Society of America

**ITFAR:** Interagency Task Force on Antimicrobial Resistance

**JCAHO:** Joint Commission on Accreditation of Health care Organizations

**MRSA:** methicillin-resistant *Staphylococcus aureus*

**MSSA:** methicillin-sensitive *Staphylococcus aureus*

**NHII:** National Health Information Infrastructure

**NIH:** National Institutes of Health

**NME:** new molecular entity

**NNIS:** National Nosocomial Infection Surveillance

**PD:** pharmacodynamic

**PDUFA:** Prescription Drug User Fee Acts

**PHC4:** Pennsylvania Health Care Cost Containment Commission

**PK:** pharmacokinetic

**QAPI:** Quality Assessment and Performance Improvement

**QIO:** quality improvement organization

**SHEA:** Society for Health care Epidemiology of America

**TB:** tuberculosis

**VRE:** vancomycin-resistant enterococci

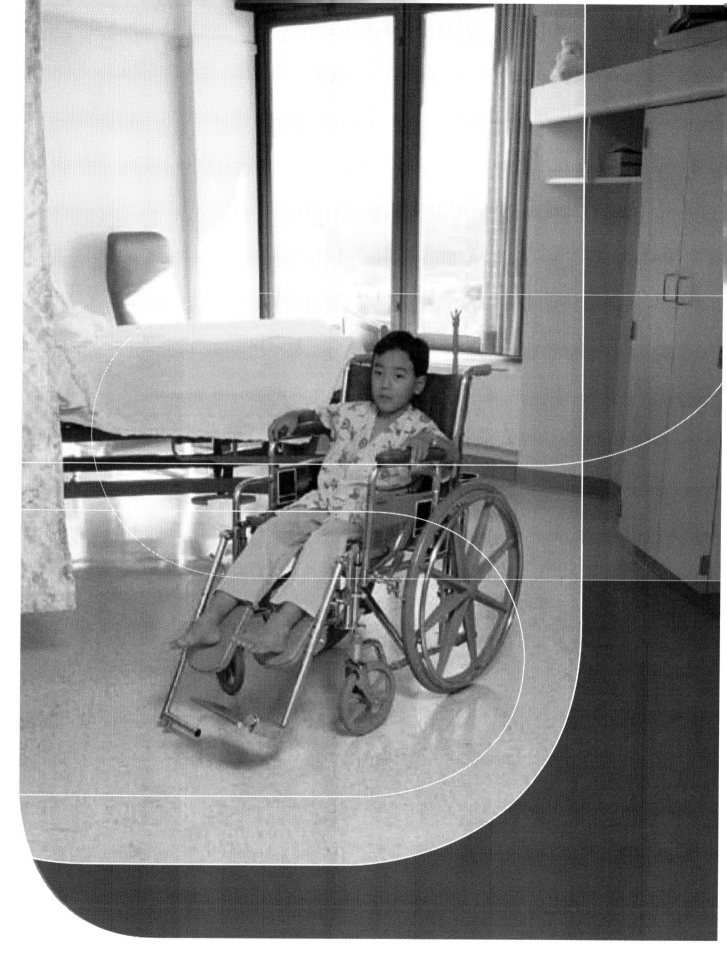

# Biographies

## Advisory Committee

**KENNETH J. ARROW** (Chair) is Professor of Economics (Emeritus) at Stanford University. He began his academic career as a research associate in the Cowles Commission for Research in Economics (1947–1949) and assistant professor of economics at the University of Chicago (1948–1949). From 1949 to 1968, he served on the faculty at Stanford University, eventually becoming a professor of economics, statistics, and operations research. From 1968 to 1979, he was at Harvard University, as a professor of economics and as James Bryant Conant University Professor. He then returned to Stanford, as Joan Kenney Professor of Economics and Professor of Operations Research, retiring in 1991.

Arrow has been a consultant to the RAND Corporation since 1948, was a staff member of the President's Council of Economic Advisers in 1962, and has served as a member and officer of numerous academic societies, including president of the Econometric Society, the American Economic Association, the International Economic Association, the International Society for Inventory Research, and the Society for Social Choice and Welfare. He has received several awards, including the Nobel Memorial Prize in Economic Science in 1972.

He received his doctorate in economics and master's in mathematics from Columbia University.

**DONALD KENNEDY** is President Emeritus, Bing Professor of Environmental Science and Policy Emeritus, and a Senior Fellow of the Institute for International Studies at Stanford University. His current research interests include interdisciplinary studies on the development of policies regarding such transboundary environmental problems as major land-use changes, economically driven alterations in agricultural practice, global climate change, and the development of regulatory policies. He served as president of the university from 1980 to 1992 and oversaw the introduction of the environmental policy quarter at Stanford's center in Washington, D.C., in 1993. He was commissioner of the U.S. Food and Drug Administration from 1977 to 1979.

Kennedy is currently the editor-in-chief of *Science*, director of the Carnegie Endowment for International Peace, and Co-chair of the National Academies' Project on Science, Technology and Law. He is also a member of the National Academy of Sciences, the American Academy of Arts and Sciences, and the American Philosophical Society.

He received a doctorate in biology from Harvard University.

**SIMON A. LEVIN** is Moffett Professor of Biology at Princeton and the director of the university's Center for BioComplexity. His principal research interests are in understanding how macroscopic patterns and processes are maintained at the level of ecosystems and the biosphere, in terms of ecological and evolutionary mechanisms that operate primarily at the level of organisms. Much of his work concerns the evolution of diversification, the mechanisms sustaining biological diversity in natural systems, and the implications for ecosystem structure and functioning. He has done much work on the modeling of epidemiological dynamics, including antibiotic resistance.

Levin is a member of the National Academy of Sciences and the American Philosophical Society, as well as a fellow with the American Academy of Arts and Sciences and the American Association for the Advancement of Science. Levin received the MacArthur Award from the Ecological Society of America and its Distinguished Service Award, the Okubo Prize from the Society for Mathematical Biology and the Japanese Society for Theoretical Biology, the 2004 Heineken Prize for Environmental Sciences from the Royal Netherlands Academy of Arts and Sciences, and the 2005 Kyoto Prize for Basic Sciences.

**SAUL LEVMORE,** Dean and William B. Graham Professor of Law at University of Chicago, has taught courses and written in torts, corporations, nonprofit organizations, comparative law, public choice, corporate tax, commercial law, insurance, and contracts. Prior to joining the University of Chicago, Levmore served on the faculty at the University of Virginia, where he was the Brokaw Professor of Corporate Law, the Albert Clark Tate, Jr. Research Professor, and the Class of 1962 and Barron F. Black Research Professor. Levmore is also the president of the American Law Deans Association and a member of the American Academy of Arts and Sciences.

He received his law degree as well as a Ph.D. in economics at Yale University and an honorary LL.D from IIT Chicago-Kent Law School.

**JOHN E. MCGOWAN, JR.,** is Professor of Epidemiology, Medicine (Infectious Diseases), and Pathology and Laboratory Medicine and Director of the MD/MPH program at Emory University's School of Medicine and Rollins School of Public Health. His research interests include antimicrobial resistance and usage practices; the relationship of antimicrobial use and resistance epidemiology and mechanisms of antimicrobial resistance, especially those associated with health care settings; and infectious disease epidemiology. He is a fellow of the American Academy of Microbiology, the American College of Epidemiology, and the Infectious Diseases Society of America. He is also an adviser to the Clinical and Laboratory Standards Institute (formerly the National Committee for Clinical Laboratory Standards) and has served on other U.S. committees concerned with infectious diseases. He formerly served as Chair of the Microbial Devices Review Panel for the FDA.

McGowan is a member of several journal editorial boards, including *Infection Control* and *Hospital Epidemiology* and *Emerging Infectious Diseases.* He has published widely in the medical literature on the topics of antimicrobial resistance and its relationship to antimicrobial use.

He received a bachelor's degree from Dartmouth and his MD degree from Harvard University.

## Research Team

**RAMANAN LAXMINARAYAN** is a Senior Fellow at Resources for the Future in Washington, D.C. His research deals with the integration of epidemiological models of infectious disease and the economic analysis of public health problems. He has worked with the World Health Organization on evaluating malaria treatment policy in Africa and has served on an Institute of Medicine Committee on the Economics of Antimalarial Drugs. He teaches at Johns Hopkins University and Princeton University. Laxminarayan received his undergraduate degree in engineering from the Birla Institute of Technology and Science in Pilani, India, and both his master's degree in public health and his doctorate in economics are from the University of Washington, Seattle.

**ANUP MALANI** is a Professor of Law at the University of Chicago. He is also a Research Affiliate for the Joint Center for Poverty Research at Northwestern University and the University of Chicago. Malani teaches, among other classes, Health Law, Corporations, and Bankruptcy. His research examines the control of infectious disease, placebo effects, antibiotic resistance, medical malpractice liability, and the conduct of and inferences from medical trials. He graduated from the University of Chicago Law School in 2000. He clerked for the Hon. Stephen F. Williams, U.S. Court of Appeals for the D.C. Circuit in 2000–2001 and for U.S. Supreme Court Justice Sandra Day O'Connor in 2001–

2002. Malani received a Ph.D. from the University of Chicago's Deparment of Economics in 2003. Between 2002 and 2006, He was an Associate Professor at the University of Virginia Law School and the Health Evaluation Sciences Department of the University of Virginia Medical School.

**DAVID HOWARD** is an Assistant Professor in the Rollins School of Public Health at Emory University. His research focuses on using economics and statistics to better understand physician decisionmaking and its implications for public policy. Currently Howard is studying trends in treated disease prevalence and the value of cancer screening in patients with limited life expectancy. He is also examining the impact of quality on patients' choice of hospital for kidney transplantation. He has acted as an adviser or consultant to the American Cancer Society, the Division of Transplantation in the Department of Health and Human Services, and the Institute of Medicine. He received his doctorate from the economics track of the health policy program at Harvard University in 2000.

**DAVID L. SMITH** is a scientist at the Division of Epidemiology and Population Studies at the Fogarty International Center, National Institutes of Health. His research interests include mathematical epidemiology and economic epidemiology; academic subdisciplines that use mathematical models to understand the epidemiology, ecology, population dynamics, and control of infectious diseases; and the interplay between the biology of infectious diseases, economics, and human behavior. He has published on the economic impact of agricultural antibiotic use, the spatial spread and economic epidemiology of hospital-acquired pathogens, the epidemiology of malaria, and the spatial spread of raccoon rabies. He earned doctoral and master's degrees from Princeton University in ecology and evolutionary biology, and master's and undergraduate degrees from Brigham Young University in mathematics.

Smith conducted research for this report as a part of his official duties at the Fogarty International Center, NIH.

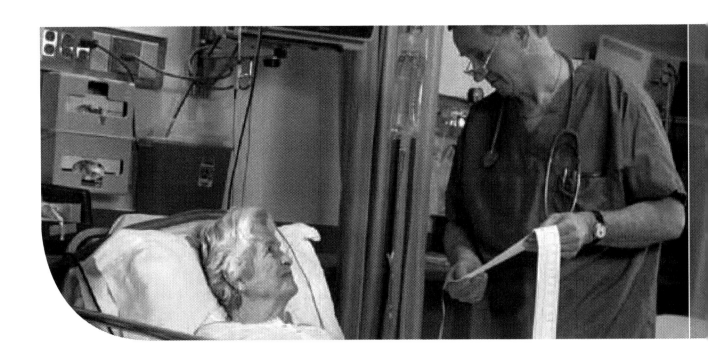

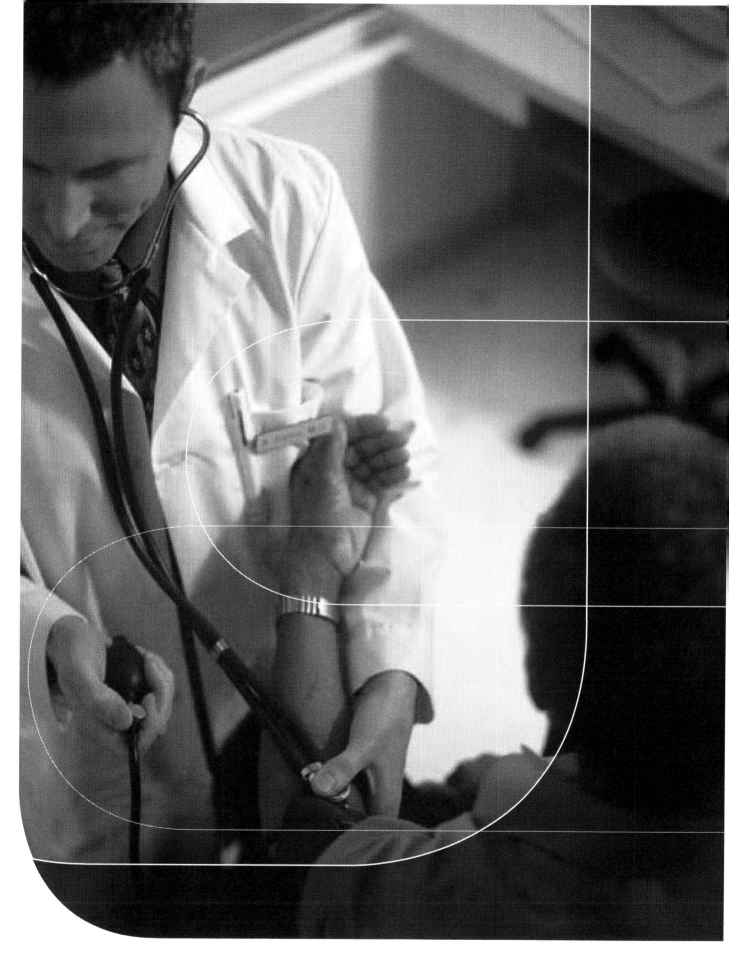

# Consultation Participants

**MR. GREGORY ANDERSON**
Centers for Disease Control and Prevention

**MS. ALISON AYERS**
Commercial Head, Infectious Disease
Pfizer, Inc.

**DR. BILL BAINE**
Agency for Health care Research and Quality

**DR. JOHN BARTLETT**
Chief, Division of Infectious Diseases
Johns Hopkins University Medical School

**DR. SUSAN BERGER**
Director, Science Knowledge and Policy
Pfizer, Inc.

**DR. MARTIN BLASER**
Professor of Internal Medicine
Chair, Department of Medicine
New York University and Infectious Diseases Society
of America

**DR. MACIEK BONI**
Stanford Genome Technology Center

**DR. PATRICIA BRADFORD**
Associate Director, Infectious Diseases
Wyeth Research

**DR. EDDY BRESNITZ**
Deputy Commissioner and Chief Epidemiologist
New Jersey Department of Health and Senior Services

**MR. MARK BRUECKL**
Pharmacy Affairs Manager
Academy of Managed Care Pharmacy

**PROFESSOR TIM BUCHMAN**
Harry Edison Professor of Surgery
Washington University School of Medicine

**DR. KAREN BUSH**
Pre-clinical Anti-Infectives Team Leader
Johnson & Johnson Pharmaceutical Research & Development

**DR. BARRY EISENSTEIN**
Senior Vice President of Scientific Affairs
Cubist Pharmaceuticals

**DR. SIMON ELLIOTT**
Registered Patent Agent
Foley & Lardner LLP

**DR. CAROLYN FISCHER**
Senior Fellow
Resources for the Future

**PROFESSOR NEIL FISHMAN**
Associate Professor of Medicine
University of Pennsylvania Medical School

**PROFESSOR LOUIS GARRISON**
University of Washington

**DR. KAREN GERLACH**
Senior Program Officer
Robert Wood Johnson Foundation

**DR. ROSEMARY GIBSON**
Senior Program Officer
Robert Wood Johnson Foundation

**DR. DON GOLDMANN**
Senior Vice President
Institute for Health care Improvement

**DR. ROBERT GREGORY**
Northeast Regional Pharmacy Director
Aetna U.S. Health care, Inc.

**DR. PETER GROSS**
Hackensack University Medical Center and Infectious Diseases
Society of America

**MR. ROBERT GUIDOS**
Director, Policy and Government Relations
Infectious Diseases Society of America

**MS. JULIE HANTMAN**
Program Officer, Public Health and Science
Infectious Diseases Society of America

**MS. ALINE HOLMES**
Senior Vice President, Clinical Affairs
New Jersey Hospital Association

**DR. THOMAS HOOTON**
Director, Center for Women's Health
University of Miami

**PROFESSOR DAVID HYMAN**
University of Illinois

**MS. SUSAN JENNINGS**
U.S. Environmental Protection Agency

**DR. LUTHER LINDER**
Director, Public Health Laboratory Services
U.S. Department of Defense

**PROFESSOR JOHN MCGOWAN**
Rollins School of Public Health
Emory University

**MR. PAUL MILLER**
Research Head, Antibacterials
Pfizer, Inc.

**MS. TESSA MILOFSKY**
U.S. Environmental Protection Agency

**DR. TRISH PERL**
Associate Professor of Medicine
Johns Hopkins Medical Institutions

**DR. KENT PETERS**
Program Officer, Antibacterial Resistance
NIAID/NIH/DHHS Bacteriology and Mycology Branch

**PROFESSOR TOMAS PHILIPSON**
University of Chicago Law School
Harris School of Public Policy Studies

**PROFESSOR RON POLK**
Chair, Department of Pharmacy
Virginia Commonwealth University and Medical
College of Virginia

**DR. JOHN POWERS**
Lead Medical Officer, Antimicrobial Drug Development
and Resistance Initiatives
U.S. Food and Drug Administration

**DR. CHESLEY RICHARDS**
Division of Health care Quality Promotion
Centers for Disease Control and Prevention

**DR. AMIRA ROESS**
Science Director
National Commission on Industrial Farm Animal
Production in the United States

**DR. BARBARA RUDOLPH**
Director, Leaps and Measures
The Leapfrog Group

**DR. DAN SAHM**
Chief Scientific Officer
Focus Diagnostics

**MS. MARISSA SCHLAIFER**
Pharmacy Affairs Director
Academy of Managed Care Pharmacy

**DR. DAVID SCHWARTZ**
Senior Physician
Stroger Hospital of Cook County

**DR. MICHAEL STRAMPEL**
Clinical Program Manager
Blue Cross Blue Shield of Michigan

**DR. TODD WEBER**
Director, Office of Antimicrobial Resistance
Centers for Disease Control and Prevention

**DR. DAVID WHITE**
U.S. Food and Drug Administration

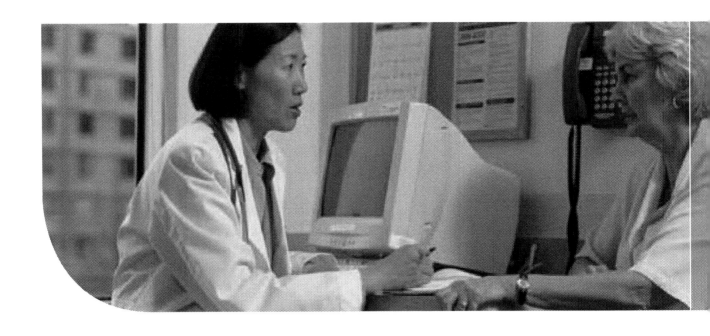

For Product Safety Concerns and Information please contact our EU
representative  GPSR@taylorandfrancis.com
Taylor & Francis Verlag GmbH, Kaufingerstraße 24, 80331 München, Germany

www.ingramcontent.com/pod-product-compliance
Ingram Content Group UK Ltd.
Pitfield, Milton Keynes, MK11 3LW, UK
UKHW052014180425
457613UK00025B/1285